MEDICAL AND BIOLOGICAL IMAGE ANALYSIS

Edited by **Robert Koprowski**

Medical and Biological Image Analysis http://dx.doi.org/10.5772/intechopen.72065 Edited by Robert Koprowski

Part of IntechOpen Book Series: Biomedical Engineering, Volume 1
Book Series Editor: Robert Koprowski

Contributors

K.S Tamilselvan, G Murugesan, Stephane Avril, Sareh Behdadfar, Laurent Navarro, Mary M Maleckar, Hans Henrik Odland, Joakim Sundnes, Francisco Mesa-Linares, Abdelkader Moumen, Ester Zumpano, Pietro Cinaglia, Luciano Caroprese, Giueppe Lucio Cascini, Francesco Dattola, Pasquale Iaquinta, Miriam Iusi, Pierangelo Veltri, Zisheng Li, Peifei Zhu, Takashi Toyomura, Yoshimi Noguchi, Hemalatha R.J, Thamizhvani T.R, Josephin Arockia Dhivya A, Josline Elsa Joseph, Bincy Babu, Chandrasekaran R

First published in London, United Kingdom, 2018 by IntechOpen
IntechOpen is the global imprint of INTECHOPEN LIMITED, registered in England and Wales, registration number: 11086078, The Shard, 25th floor, 32 London Bridge Street
London, SE19SG – United Kingdom
Printed in Croatia

British Library Cataloguing-in-Publication Data
A catalogue record for this book is available from the British Library

Additional hard copies can be obtained from orders@intechopen.com

Medical and Biological Image Analysis, Edited by Robert Koprowski
p. cm.
Print ISBN 978-1-78923-330-8
Online ISBN 978-1-78923-331-5

For EU product safety concerns:
IN TECH d.o.o., Prolaz Marije Krucifikse Kozulić 3, 51000 Rijeka, Croatia,
info@intechopen.com or visit our website at intechopen.com.

IntechOpen Book Series
Biomedical Engineering

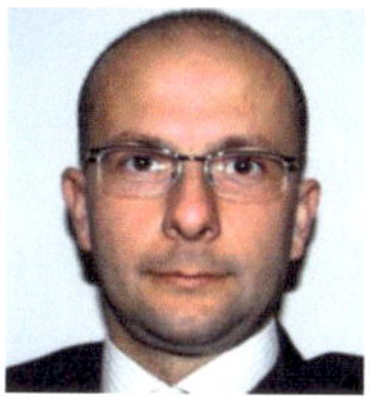

Robert Koprowski 1997 earned a Master of Science degree in electrical engineering and metrology. After graduation, he started working as an assistant at the Faculty of Technology (now the Faculty of Computer Science and Materials Science) of the University of Silesia. His interests have been focused on the issues of biomedical image analysis and processing, which in 2003 resulted in defending his doctoral dissertation on the use of image analysis and processing in medicine (in scoliosis) at the Faculty of Automatic Control, Electronics and Computer Science of the Silesian University of Technology in Gliwice. Dr. Koprowski is an author of more than 140 publications and is currently affiliated with the University of Silesia in Katowice.

Book Series Editor and Editor of Volume 1:
Robert Koprowski
University of Silesia, Poland

Scope of the Series

Biomedical engineering is one of the fastest growing interdisciplinary branches of science and industry. The combination of electronics and computer science with biology and medicine has resulted in improved patient diagnosis, reduced rehabilitation time and better quality of life. Nowadays, all medical imaging devices, medical instruments or new laboratory techniques are the result of the cooperation of specialists in various fields. The series of biomedical engineering books covers such areas of knowledge as chemistry, physics, electronics, medicine and biology. This series is intended for doctors, engineers and scientists involved in biomedical engineering or those wanting to start working in this field.

Contents

Preface

This book deals with medical image analysis methods. In particular, it contains two significant chapters on image segmentation as well as some selected examples of the application of image analysis and processing methods. Despite the significant development of information technology methods used in modern image analysis and processing algorithms, the segmentation process remains open. This is mainly due to intra-patient variability and/or scene diversity. Segmentation is equally difficult in the case of ultrasound imaging and depends on the location of the probe or the contact force. Regardless of the imaging method, segmentation must be tailored for a specific application in almost every case. These types of application areas for various imaging methods are included in this book. In addition to the aforementioned examples of medical image segmentation, the issues related to medical image analysis by means of other complex methods have been discussed here. I hope that the book will be popular among not only bioengineers but also computer scientists and doctors.

Robert Koprowski
University of Silesia
Sosnowiec, Poland

Section 1

Image Processing

Chapter 1

Image Segmentation

Kumaravel Subramaniam Tamilselvan and
Govindasamy Murugesan

Additional information is available at the end of the chapter

http://dx.doi.org/10.5772/intechopen.76428

Abstract

Image segmentation is one of the important and useful techniques in medical image processing. As the image segmentation technique results robust and high degree of accuracy, it is very much useful for the analysis of different image modalities, such as computerized tomography (CT) and magnetic resonance imaging (MRI) in the medical field. CT imaging gives more importance than MRI because of its wider availability, inexpensive and sensitiveness. In most cases, CT offers information needed to make decisions during urgent situations.

Keywords: computerized tomography, magnetic resonance imaging, watershed, wavelet transform, segmentation, neural network

1. Introduction

The main aim of image segmentation is to optimize the physician's diagnosis by automatically detecting the suspicious patterns and classifying the abnormalities. In order to achieve this, several methods are employed. One of which is hybrid algorithm based on wavelet transform and watershed segmentation (WT-WS), used to isolate the tumor from different medical image modalities, especially from CT and MRI images. Various features like peak signal to noise ratio (PSNR), root mean square error (RMSE) and average difference (AD) can be measured to evaluate the efficiency of an algorithm.

This chapter elaborates the need for image segmentation, different types of segmentation, merits and demerits of each method and techniques to overcome the limitations of each method. Various categories of segmentation are clustering, edge detection and region extraction [1]. The main drawbacks with the conventional image segmentation techniques are over segmentation and high sensitivity to noise. To overcome these problems, image segmentation method based on the combination of wavelet transform and watershed segmentation algorithm can be employed. Over segmentation and noise problems are reduced by applying watershed technique to carry out the low pass filtered image from wavelet transform [2].

1.1. Need for image segmentation

Segmentation is an important stage of the image recognition system, because it extracts the objects of our interest, for further processing such as description or recognition. Segmentation of an image is in practice for the classification of image pixel [3]. Segmentation techniques are used to isolate the desired object from the image in order to perform analysis of the object. For example, a tumor, cancer or a block in the blood flow can be easily isolated from its background with the help of image segmentation technique [4]. Various techniques are available for the segmentation of monochrome images. The segmentation of color images is more complicated as each pixel in the color images is vector valued [5].

The existing image segmentation techniques have the limitations of over-segmentation and high sensitivity to noise. The earlier techniques frequently use the statistical methods to find those features in a complete brain MRI or CT images. Furthermore, the segmentation process takes more time for processing and some of the features are redundant and get overlapped [6]. The determination of features of the whole image is a difficult task too. Due to the presence of redundant and overlapped features, an accurate result cannot be obtained. These methods make use of both statistical and non-statistical features. For example, in the neural network-based segmentation, a neural network is first trained with statistical features and then trained with non-statistical features [7]. The two times training process of the neural network with different features gives the insignificant result [8]. Magnetic resonance imaging is an emerging field of research in medical imaging filed, which can be used to recognize the features of human brain. The main aim of research in this field is to identify and detect the abnormalities in human brain automatically [9].

2. Wavelet and watershed-based image segmentation method

The wavelet and watershed-based image segmentation method consists of three stages, namely image enhancement, image segmentation and feature extraction. In image enhancement step, the contrast level of the CT and MRI images are improved by employing wavelet-based filtering technique without distorting the sharp edges [10]. The contrast-enhanced images are then applied to watershed-based image segmentation technique. Performance measurement factors such as peak signal to noise ratio (PSNR), root mean square error (RMSE) and average difference (AD) are calculated in the feature extraction step. The extracted features are used to compare the segmentation efficiency of the present technique with other-segmentation techniques. The above mentioned image segmentation technique is illustrated in **Figure 1**.

2.1. Image enhancement

Contrast enhancement of the medical image is the technique of smoothing the image and removal of noise in the image [11]. As the noise removal is affecting the segmentation

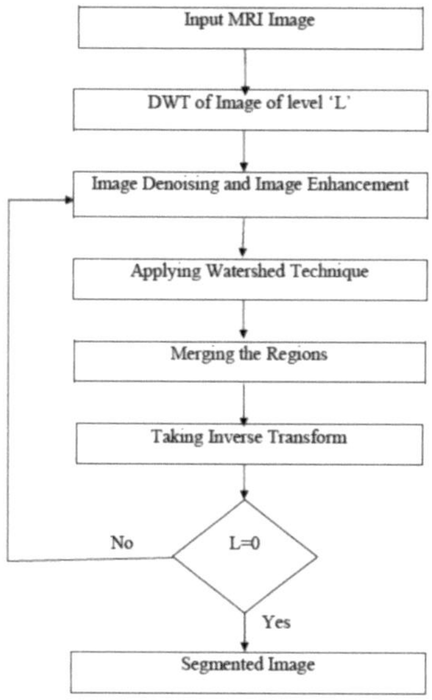

Figure 1. Block diagram wavelet transform and watershed-based image segmentation technique.

efficiency, this step is important in the image segmentation process. All the medical images contain both smoothing and detailed information. The smoothing information can be easily filtered out by using a number of morphological filters.

2.2. Wavelet decomposition

Wavelet transform decomposes the MRI image into a multiresolution representation, which consists of the low frequency approximation information and the high frequency detailed information. Given an MRI image, the multiresolution representation is generated by successive filtering using quadrature mirror filter. The basic function of a wavelet is to decompose the given image into different subbands. This can be done by using either uniform or octave band decomposition as shown in **Figure 2**.

From **Figure 2**, it is shown that, wavelet transform decompose a given image into four sub-images.

The decomposed images are,

- Low-Low(LL): Low frequency in both horizontal and vertical directions
- Low-High(LH): Low frequency in horizontal and high frequency in vertical direction
- High-Low(HL): High frequency horizontal direction and low frequency in vertical direction
- High-High(HH): High frequency in both horizontal and vertical directions

To decompose an image, filter banks are used with low pass and high pass filters.

Figure 3 shows the decomposition of an image into four sub-images.

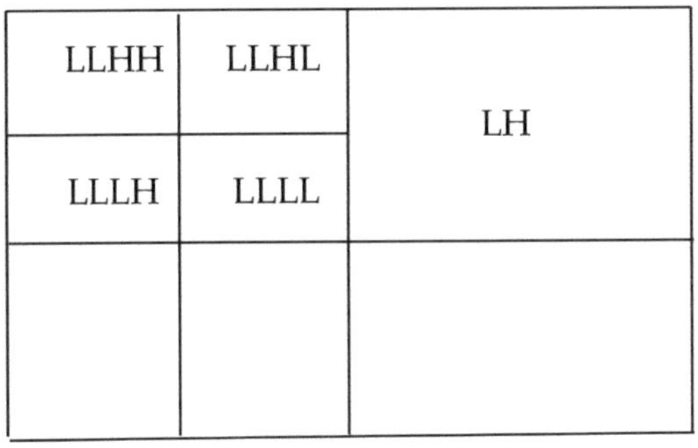

Figure 2. Two level wavelet decomposition.

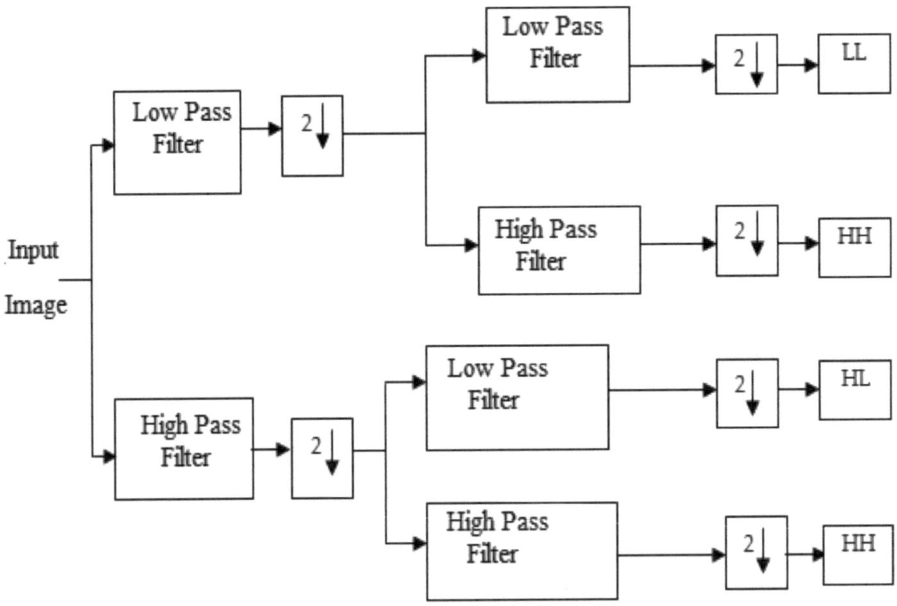

Figure 3. Four sub bands of decomposition of image.

The LL sub-image is called the approximation image, while the LH, HL and HH are called the detailed images which are illustrated in **Figure 3**. Various image processing techniques can be applied to the sub band images for different solutions. Increasing the number of decomposition produces coarse contours that may hide some relevant features of the carotid artery walls.

2.3. Pyramidal representation

Pyramidal representation of an image tends to examine an image in multi resolution methods. Different types of decomposing an image are Gaussian Pyramids, Laplacian Pyramids and wavelets. Out of the above methods, Gaussian and Laplacian Pyramid give some loss of information. But the wavelet-based decomposition will overcome these drawbacks. Haar wavelet transform can be selected for this purpose.

2.4. Steps in the Wavelet-based image enhancement

Steps to be followed when using wavelet decomposition of an image:

1. Separate the given image into LL, LH, HL and HH sub-images using a low pass filter at a scale of 2j
2. Repeat the process of decomposition on the LL sub band until the number of sub bands is equal to 4.
3. Find the J scale transforms, for the original image as represented by,

$$W^{2i}, (W_H^{2i}, W_V^{2i}, W_D^{2i})\ 1 \le i \le J \tag{1}$$

for $j = 1, 2, \ldots, J$

where W^{2i}, W_H^{2i}, W_V^{2i} and W_D^{2i} represents transform results LL, LH, HL and HH at 2^j scale, respectively. This representation is composed of a coarse signal at resolution 2^i and a set of detailed signal at resolution 2^i-2^j.

2.5. Watershed-based image segmentation

In the watershed-based image segmentation, the image is splitted into different areas. Normally watershed-based segmentation will lead to an over-segmentation of the image, especially for noisy image such as medical CT images. To avoid this oversegmentation, either the input image must be preprocessed or the different regions of the image must be merged based on similarity [12].

It is easy to understand the watershed technique by consider the image as a plain surface where high pixel values correspond to peaks and low pixel values correspond to valleys. Same as actual watersheds in irrigation, if a drop of water falls on any particular point of the contour, automatically it will flow to lower ground till it reaches a local minimum which is catchment basin and the collected points in a particular basin is called as a member of that watershed. Expressions (2) and (3) represent the watershed transform.

AS a first step, we have to calculate the local gradients within a particular image Let the original image is 'I' and 'G' is a low variance Gaussian Kernel. The blurred gradient 'B' can be represented as in the expression (2).

$$B = G * \nabla I \tag{2}$$

where ∇I is defined such that

$$\nabla I(i,j) = \left[I(i,j+1) - I(i,j)\right]^2 + \left[I(i,j) - I(i+1,j)\right]^2 \tag{3}$$

The next step is to find the local minima of **B**. An element m(i, j) is said to be a local minimum if $m(i,j) < p(i_0, j_0) \forall (i_0, j_0) \in N(i,j)$ where N(i,j) represents spatial neighborhood of the element at row i and column j in eight connectivity. The local minima m_i represent the catchment basins of the image and are each assigned with a unique label greater than zero. The final step is to follow each element in B toward its lowest valued neighbor until it merges into one of the catchment basins m_i. Eqs. (4) and (5) give the watershed and an edge map equation respectively. Once an element merges with catchment basin m_i, it assumes the label of that basin. The above function can be represented as WS. So the watershed W is defined as in the Eq. (4).

$$W = WS\left(G^{*} \nabla\ I\right) \tag{4}$$

The resulting edge map E is defined in the expression (5).

$$E(i,j) = \begin{cases} 1 & \nabla W(i,j) > 0 \\ 0 & Otherwise \end{cases} \tag{5}$$

where W (i,j) is the label of watershed in which element (i,j) is a member after all of the watersheds have been labeled.

2.6. Limitations of watershed transform-based image segmentation

Noise is a great challenge in the segmentation process of an image with watershed-based technique and over segmentation is another important drawback with watershed-based image segmentation. These drawbacks can be avoided by using region merging method. A combination of wavelet and watershed-based image segmentation method can also be used to address the above problems.

2.7. Steps of the watershed algorithm-based image segmentation

STEP 1: Read the original image (I0).

STEP 2: Take L level wavelet transform of image (IL).

STEP 3: Smooth the image and remove noise particles using wavelet denoising.

STEP 4: Apply watershed segmentation.

STEP 5: Resulting merged region image is projected onto the IL-1 layer by an Inverse wavelet transform.

STEP 6: Go to step3 and repeat the above procedure until L equals 0 (initial stage).

Acquisition the source image: Get the MRI image, which is the source image for the segmentation process obtained from a clinic.

Contrast maximization: maximization of contrast of an image is adopted to identify and minimize number of valley points. Wavelet transform is preferred for contrast enhancement.

To maximize the contrast, first compute $\alpha_{n,s}$ using the Eq. (6) and (7).

Let n be the decomposition level,

http://dx.doi.org/10.5772/intechopen.76428

$$E_{n,s} = \frac{\sum_{i,j} \mid x_{,,s}(x, j) \mid}{N} \tag{6}$$

$$\alpha_{n,s} = \frac{En + 1, s}{\sum_s En + 1, s/3} \tag{7}$$

where s is the sub band which indicates LH, HL and HH. $E_{n,s}$ is the average absolute value of a specific sub band *s* in level *n*. N is the number of coefficients of each sub band. $\bar{x}_{n,s}(i,j)$ is enhanced sub band from each sub band $x_{n,s}(i,j)$ and can be computed by Eq. (8).

$$x_{n,s}(\mathrm{i}, \mathrm{j}) = \alpha_{n,s} x_{n,s}(i, j) \tag{8}$$

Enhanced image is computed for each sub band and reconstructed the image using inverse wavelet transform. Resulting image is the contrast-enhanced image.

Conversion of objects of interest: the watershed transform detects intensity valleys in the image. The enhanced image is converted into the objects of interest with high intensity valleys.

Detection of intensity valleys: all the intensity valleys are below a particular threshold. The location rather than the size of the regions is important. The min function modifies the image to contain only those valleys found by the extended min function. The min function will also change a valleys pixel value to zero (deepest possible valley for unit 8 images). All regions containing an imposed minimum will be detected by the watershed transform.

Watershed segmentation: watershed segmentation of the imposed minima image is accomplished with the watershed function. The watershed function returns a label matrix containing non-negative numbers that correspond to watershed regions. Pixels that do not fall into any watershed region are given a pixel value of zero.

However, the image is degraded by noise and so cause over-segmentation. Therefore over-segmentation images are further merged in some regions. The region to be merged is based on homogeneity and similarity criteria based on the wavelet coefficients. Mean, second- and third-order central moments values of the wavelet coefficients of each of the regions are calculated.

Merging over-segmentation regions: The watershed transform is sensitive to the change of the data therefore the noise objective brim and then changes inside objectives can lead to over-segmentation. Over segmentation is caused by the watershed transform, and the image background is divided into several parts and merged using the following conditions:

a. The regions that will be combined are neighbors.

b. The characteristics of the region, which will be combined, should be similar.

c. The big region after combining is useful.

The regions which are neighbors and similar pixel values can be combined. After combination, the background and the target image are separated. Usually, similitude can be defined according to gray, texture, and so on.

If Bi is set of boundary points of catchment basin I (CBi), Ni is the number of Bi, then the definition of B mean (i) is given by the Eq. (9).

$$B\ mean\ (i) = f(pj)/Ni \tag{9}$$

During projection from Ith layer to (I-1)th layer, a parent-child spatial relationship between the image elements of two successive layers is defined. This relationship is evaluated by means of a similarity measure. The children of a layer may belong to different parents in the upper layer. The similarity between a child image element and its possible parents describes the similarities.

3. Feature extraction and segmentation quality evaluation

The feature extraction is mainly done in evaluating the quality and efficiency of the proposed image segmentation algorithm. The different parameters such as root mean square error (RMSE), peak signal to noise ratio (PSNR) and average difference (AD) are used to measure the performance of the resultant segmented image of different techniques and compared with that of the proposed algorithm.

3.1. Root mean square error (RMSE)

RMSE is used to measure the difference between the source image and the segmented image, the smaller the value of RMSE, the better the segmentation performance. Mathematical representation of RMSE is given in Eq. (10).

$$\mathrm{RMSE} = \sqrt{\frac{\sum_{i=1}^{M}\sum_{j=1}^{N}[\mathrm{M(i,j)}-\mathrm{F(i,j)}]^2}{\mathrm{MxN}}} \tag{10}$$

where M and N are size of the image, *i* and *j* are the pixel positions in the image. M(i,j) is the segmented image and F(i,j) is the original image.

3.2. Peak signal to noise ratio (PSNR)

PSNR is the ratio between the maximum value of an image and the value of background noise. In terms of RMSE, PSNR is given in the Eq. (11).

$$PSNR = 10^{\times} ln\,(f_{max}/RMSE)^2 \tag{11}$$

where f_{max} is the maximum value of pixels in the segmented image. The larger the PSNR value, better the segmentation performance.

3.3. Average difference (AD)

Average difference is the difference in each pixel value between the input source image and the segmented image. Lower value of AD shows better segmentation performance.

The average difference between segmented image (f) and reference image (r) is given by the expression (12).

$$D_A = \frac{1}{MN}\sum_{i=1}^{M}\sum_{j=1}^{N}\left(| r(x,y)_{ij} - f(x,y)_{ij} | \right) \tag{12}$$

4. Sample results and discussion

This section demonstrates the performance of the proposed image segmentation algorithm for isolating the tumor part in the clinical MRI image.

The sample of normal and abnormal MRI images obtained from Kovai Medical Centre Hospital, Coimbatore, Tamil Nadu, India is illustrated in the **Figure 4**.

Segmentation algorithm is tested with MatLab tool and the simulation results are analyzed in this section. **Figures 5(a)** and **6(a)** shows the input MRI images which are the source images for segmentation. As the source images have a low contrast level, they are enhanced with wavelet transform and the resulting contrast-enhanced images are shown in **Figures 5(b)** and **6(b)**. This step is also known as preprocessing step of image segmentation.

The contrast-enhanced MRI images are then subjected to second level decomposition using wavelet transforms. They are shown in **Figures 5(c)** and **6(c)**. In this step, the high frequency terms (H terms) in the images which are identified as noise terms are separated from the image and the low frequency (L terms) terms which are identified as a region of interest. The first level decomposition produces HH, HL, LH and LL sub images. The second level decomposition produces HHHH, HHHL, LLHL and LLLL.

The decomposed images with LL term are applied to watershed segmentation process, where the boundary of the LL images has extracted to isolate the tumor from its background. This is shown in the **Figures 5(d)** and **6(d)**. The extracted boundary of the images is superimposed on first level decomposed image (LL) which is shown in the **Figures 5(e)** and **6(e)**. Boundary extractions of synthesized images by the watershed algorithm are shown in

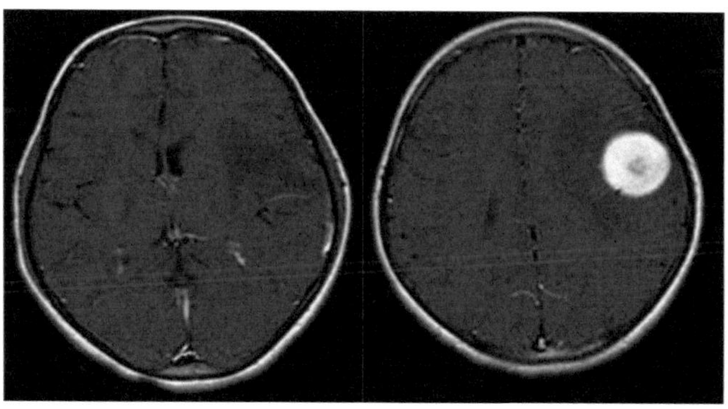

Figure 4. Sample normal and abnormal clinical MRI images.

the **Figures 5(f)** and **6(f)**. The boundaries are superimposed on the original images as shown in **Figures 5(g)** and **6(g)**.

The performance values for different types of image segmentation techniques are analyzed. From the analysis, it is evident that, the RMS error of the proposed image segmentation technique is 0.0154 which is minimum compared with other segmentation techniques (0.0236 for wavelet alone and 0.0312 for watershed alone). The value of RMSE should be minimum for an efficient segmentation technique.

The PSNR value obtained for the hybrid technique is 55.498 which is higher value than the existing techniques. The measured PSNR value is 55.416 for wavelet alone and 55.434 for watershed alone. For an efficient segmentation technique, the PSNR value should be maximum.

The average difference (AD) is the difference in each pixel value between the input source image and the segmented image. From the analysis, the value of AD of the hybrid method is 2.3611e-004 and that of the wavelet and watershed alone are 5.714e-004 and 9.725e-004, respectively. This shows that the hybrid method has a minimum value of AD compared with other segmentation techniques. Lower the value of AD, the better the segmentation performance.

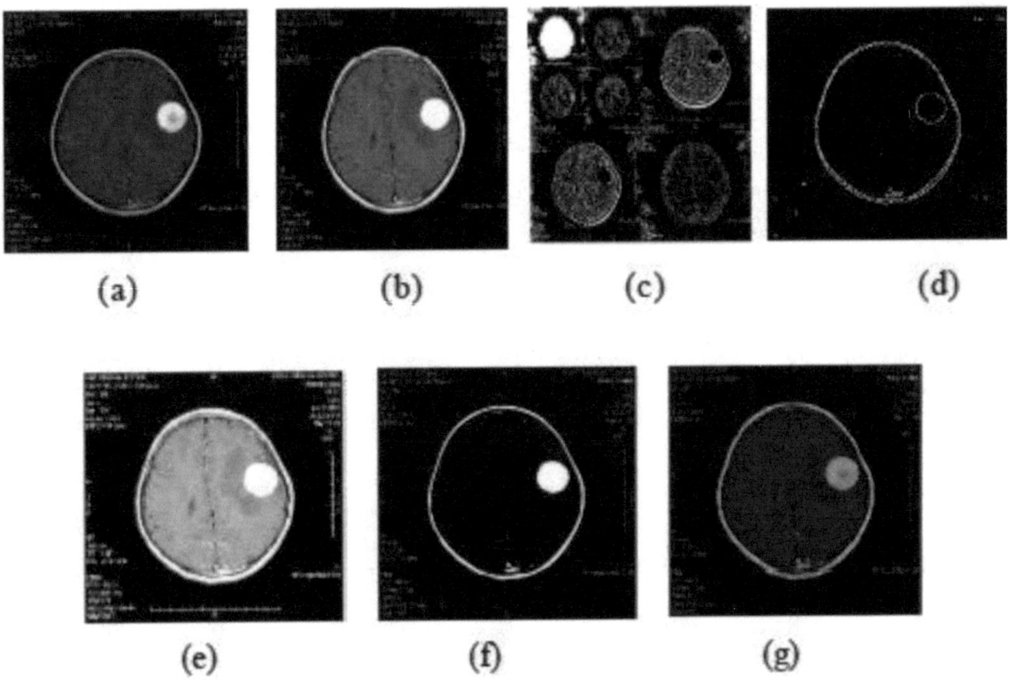

Figure 5. Simulation results for brain MRI image segmentation: (a) original MRI image (b) enhanced image (c) two level decomposition of enhanced image (d) boundary extraction of LL image using a watershed algorithm (e) boundary superimposed on first level decomposed image (LL) (f) boundary extraction of reconstructed image using a watershed algorithm (g) boundary superimposed on the original image.

http://dx.doi.org/10.5772/intechopen.76428

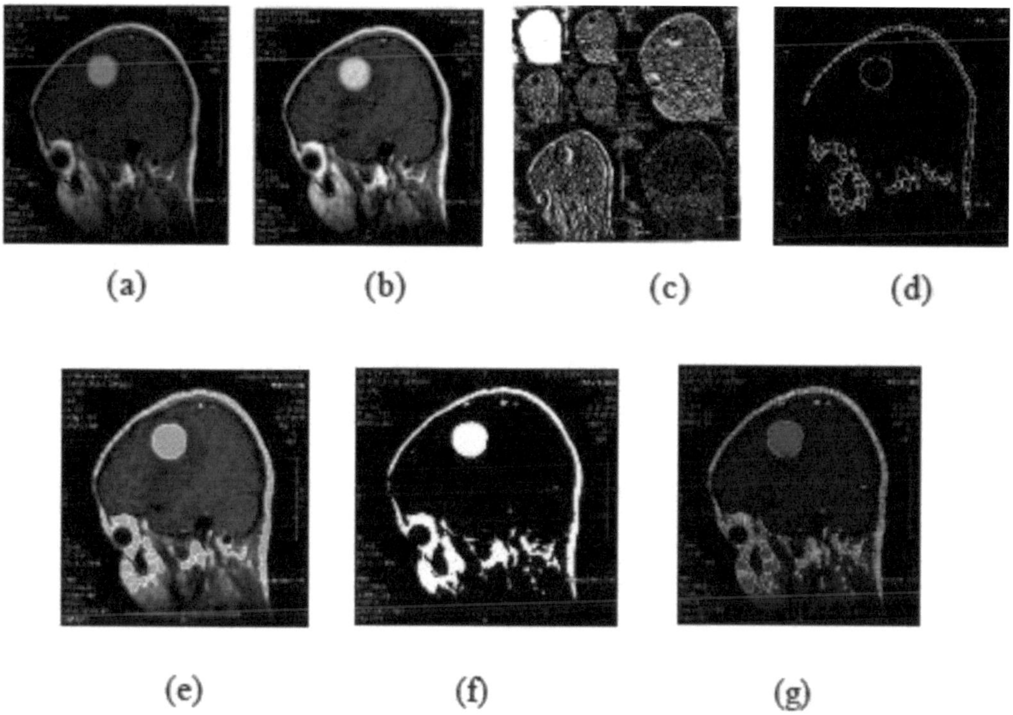

Figure 6. Simulation results for head MRI image segmentation: (a) original MRI image 2 (b) enhanced image (c) two level decomposition of enhanced image (d) boundary extraction of LL image using a watershed algorithm (e) boundary superimposed on first level decomposed image (LL) (f) boundary extraction of reconstructed image using a watershed algorithm (g) boundary superimposed on the original image.

It is inferred from the above analysis and discussion that by considering the values of performance factors, the hybrid image segmentation method which includes the wavelet and watershed method performs better than the other existing techniques.

Figure 7(a) shows the comparative chart of RMSE for proposed segmentation technique with that of other existing techniques. From the chart, it is clear that the RMSE value of the proposed technique is the minimum which ensures that the proposed segmentation technique performs well. **Figure 7(b)** illustrates the comparison of PSNR for the proposed method with existing techniques, which also prove that the proposed system in terms of PSNR is better than the other techniques. The average difference in each pixel value between the input source image and the segmented image is given in the **Figure 7(c)**. It shows that the value of AD is comparatively minimum for the proposed method. For an efficient segmentation technique, the value of average difference should be minimum. Therefore, from the simulation results and from the observation of performance measurement factors, it is evident that the proposed image segmentation algorithm which comprises of wavelet transform and watershed segmentation performs better.

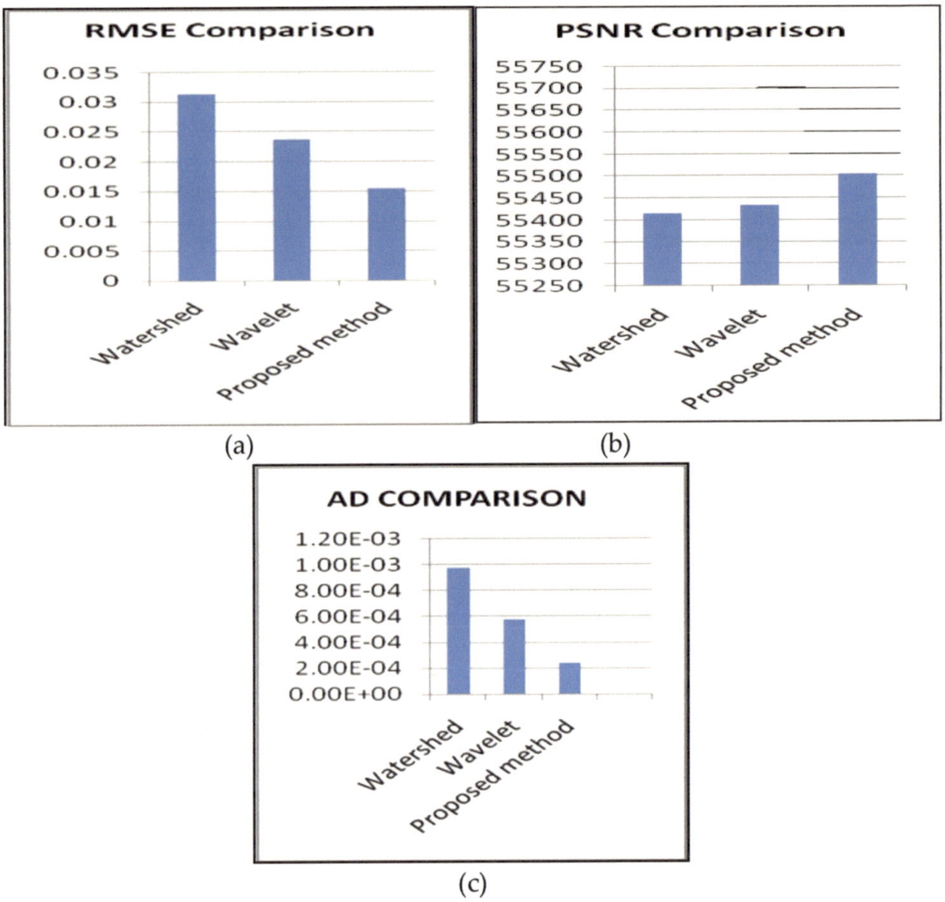

Figure 7. Comparison of performance measurement parameters for different image segmentation techniques: (a) comparison of RMSE (b) comparison of PSNR (c) comparison of average difference.

5. Conclusion of the chapter

A new segmentation technique by combining wavelet transform and watershed algorithm is proposed in this section to detect the tumor in human brain. The existing method of tumor extraction is concentrated on wavelet transform or watershed transform. But the existing techniques have a drawback of over-segmentation due to noise. The hybrid segmentation method is a multiresolution technique for image segmentation and it can be achieved without any loss of any edge information in the image. Initially, we have to choose the required resolution level of the image according to the size and number of connected objects in the image. It is also described that how regions are projected onto lower layer and build hierarchical parent-child regions relationship of successive two layers.

http://dx.doi.org/10.5772/intechopen.76428

Author details

Kumaravel Subramaniam Tamilselvan* and Govindasamy Murugesan

*Address all correspondence to: kstamilselvan@gmail.com

Kongu Engineering College, Anna University, Perundurai, India

References

[1] Chawla M, Sharma S, Jayanthi S, Kishore LT. A method for automatic detection & classification of stroke from brain CT images. In: Proceedings of IEEE Engineering in Medicine and Biology Society Conference; 2009

[2] Qurat-Ul-Ain, Latif G, Kazmi SB, Jaffar A, Anwar Mirza M. Classification and segmentation of brain tumor using texture analysis. In: International Conference on Recent Advances in Artificial Intelligence, Knowledge Engineering and Databases; 2011. pp. 147-155

[3] Cai WL, Chen SC, Zhang DQ. Fast and robust fuzzy C-means clustering algorithms incorporating local information for image segmentation. Pattern Recognition Journal. 2007;**40**(3):825-838

[4] Gadpayle P, Mahajani PS. Detection and classification of brain tumor in MRI images. International Journal of Emerging Trends in Electrical & Electronics. 2013;**5**(1):45-49

[5] Aggarwal P, Vig R, Bhadoria S, Dethe CG. Role of segmentation in medical imaging: A comparative study. International Journal of Computer Applications. 2011;**29**(1):55-64

[6] Postma GJ, Luts J, Idema AJ, Julia-Sape M, Moreno-Torres A, Gajewicz W, Suykens JAK, Heerschap A, Huffel SV, Buydens LMC. On the relevance of automatically selected single-voxel MRS and multimodal MRI and MRSI features for brain tumor differentiation. Journal of Computers in Biology and Medicine. 2011;**41**:87-97

[7] Somasundaram K, Kalaiselvi T. Fully automatic method to identify abnormal MRI head scans using fuzzy segmentation and fuzzy symmetric measure. ICGST-GVIP Journal. 2010;**10**(3):1-9

[8] Rajapakse JC, Giedd JN, Rapoport JL. Statistical approach to segmentation of single-channel cerebral MR images. IEEE Transactions on Medical Imaging. 1997;**16**(2):176-186

[9] Castellani U, Perina A, Murino V, Bellani M, Rambaldelli G, Tansella M, Brambilla P. Brain morphometry by probabilistic latent semantic analysis. In: Proceedings of the 13th International Conference on Medical Image Computing and Computer-Assisted Intervention; 2010. pp. 177-184

[10] Liu H, Chen Z, Chen X, Chen Y. Multiresolution medical image segmentation based on wavelet transform. In: Proceedings of the 2005 IEEE Engineering in Medicine and Biology 27th Annual Conference; Shanghai, China; 2005

[11] Sendur L, Selesnick IW. Bivariate shrinkage functions for wavelet-based denoising exploiting interscale dependency. IEEE Transactions on Signal Processing. 2002;**50**(11): 2744-2756

[12] Padma A, Sukanesh R. A wavelet based automatic segmentation of brain tumor in CT images using optimal statistical texture features. International Journal of Image Processing. 2011;**5**(5):552-563

Chapter 2

Active Contour Based Segmentation Techniques for Medical Image Analysis

R.J. Hemalatha, T.R. Thamizhvani,
A. Josephin Arockia Dhivya, Josline Elsa Joseph,
Bincy Babu and R. Chandrasekaran

Additional information is available at the end of the chapter

http://dx.doi.org/10.5772/intechopen.74576

Abstract

Image processing is a technique which is used to derive information from the images. Segmentation is a section of image processing for the separation or segregation of information from the required target region of the image. There are different techniques used for segmentation of pixels of interest from the image. Active contour is one of the active models in segmentation techniques, which makes use of the energy constraints and forces in the image for separation of region of interest. Active contour defines a separate boundary or curvature for the regions of target object for segmentation. The contour depends on various constraints based on which they are classified into different types such as gradient vector flow, balloon and geometric models. Active contour models are used in various image processing applications specifically in medical image processing. In medical imaging, active contours are used in segmentation of regions from different medical images such as brain CT images, MRI images of different organs, cardiac images and different images of regions in the human body. Active contours can also be used in motion tracking and stereo tracking. Thus, the active contour segmentation is used for the separation of pixels of interest for different image processing.

Keywords: energy constraints, gradient vector flow field, inflation force, geometric measures, icosahedron triangles

1. Introduction

Image processing can be defined as computerised processing of images of different types to obtain the desired output. Image processing makes use of a wide range of techniques to process the input information which is available in the form of an image. Processing of images is carried out by avoiding certain features like noise and signal distortion that affects the information present in the images. The images can be defined in different dimensions which can be used for processing. Segmentation is a part of image processing used for segregation of regions.

Segmentation is the process of separation of required information from a data for further processing. Image segmentation can be defined as the segregation of pixels of interest for effective processing. The main aim of image segmentation is to segment the meaningful regions of interest for processing. Region of interest possesses a group of pixels defined with a boundary and these may contribute to different forms such as circle, ellipse, polygon or irregular shapes. The process of segmentation does not provide information about the entire image rather associates pixel data of only the region of interest. Segmentation is a crucial process in Image analysis because it paves path for future processing of images.

In medical image analysis, segmentation is very much necessary where region of study or research is defined to a particular section of the image. If image segmentation is performed effective, the after stages of image analysis are made easier. Image segmentation provides definite and useful information or data for the high standards of automatic image analysis. Image analysis defines certain objectives for segmentation process:

- Decompose the image into parts for future analysis
- Change in representation
- Region of interest should be simple, uniform and homogenous with smooth boundary

Medical image analysis requires segmentation of images for processing of the region of interest. Different modality of images can be processed and segmented for separating the necessary pixel information. Image segmentation is described as the fundamental process in many computer vision and medical image analysis applications. With the process of segmentation, desired output from the pixels of interest is obtained.

Image segmentation can be classified into different types of algorithm based on the discontinuity and similarity of intensity values. Thresholding, region growing, region splitting, region merging, detection of boundary discontinuities (point, line and edge detection), watershed segmentation and active contours are few examples of image segmentation process. Segmentation can also be performed with the help of feature extraction process from the pixels of the image.

In this chapter, we discuss about an image segmentation technique called active contour models. These models are considered because they help in segmentation of the target object of particular data or information values from an image. Active contour technique is applied for separation of foreground from the background and the segmented region of interest undergoes further image analysis. Active contours are defined models for segmentation of pixels from the required region of interest for which processing is performed to obtain the outcome for research. Active contour models defined below are used in various different fields for image processing. Application of active contour models in medical image processing is very effective, since it separates the necessary pixels from the foreground [1].

2. Active contour models

Active contour is a type of segmentation technique which can be defined as use of energy forces and constraints for segregation of the pixels of interest from the image for further processing and analysis. Active contour described as active model for the process of segmentation. Contours are boundaries designed for the area of interest required in an image. Contour is a collection of points that undergoes interpolation process. The interpolation process can be linear, splines and polynomial which describes the curve in the image [2]. Different models of active contours are applied for the segmentation technique in image processing. The main application of active contours in image processing is to define smooth shape in the image and forms closed contour for the region. Active contour models involve snake model, gradient vector flow snake model, balloon model and geometric or geodesic contours.

Active contours can be defined as the process to obtain deformable models or structures with constraints and forces in an image for segmentation. Contour models describe the object boundaries or any other features of the image to form a parametric curve or contour. Curvature of the models is determined with various contour algorithms using external and internal forces applied. Energy functional is always associated with the curve defined in the image. External energy is defined as the combination of forces due to the image which is specifically used to control the positioning of the contour onto the image and internal energy, to control the deformable changes [3]. Constraints for a particular image in the contour segmentation depend on the requirements. The desired contour is obtained by defining the minimum of the energy functional. Deforming of the contour is described by a collection of points that finds a contour. This contour fits the required image contour defined by minimising the energy functional.

For the set of points in an image, the contour can be defined based on forces and constraints in the regions of the image. Active contours are used in various applications in the segmentation of the medical images [11, 17]. Different types of active contour models are used in various medical applications especially for the separation of required regions from the various medical images. For example, a slice of brain CT image is considered for segmentation using active contour models. The contour of the image defines the layers of the region in the brain which is shown in the **Figure 1**.

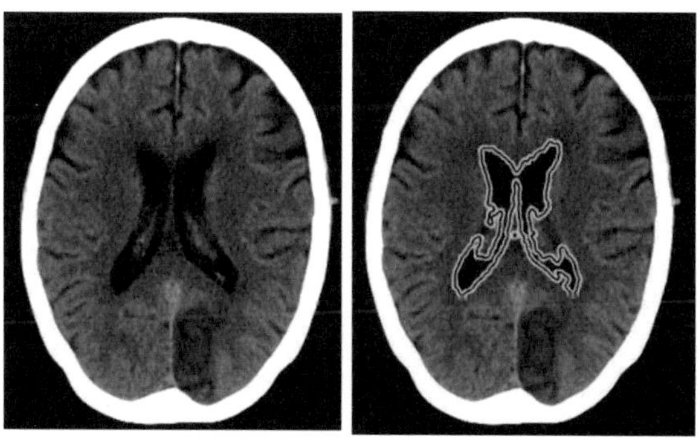

Figure 1. Segmentation of brain CT image using active contours.

Active contours can also be used for segmentation of 3-D images derived from different medical imaging modalities. 2-D slices of image data are used for the separation of target object from the 3-D images. These 2-D slices of images in all directions along with the segmented target region are subjected to 3-D reconstruction to segregate the regions. Mesh model of the 3-D image is designed before applying active contour model. The mesh helps in the formation of deformable contours of the target object in the directional 2-D slices of the 3-D images [14].

Different types of images from various 3-D imaging modalities like MRI, CT, PET, SPECT can be segmented and processed with these active contour models. The early diagnosis and detection of abnormalities in the target regions can be performed with the help of active contour models in 3-D imaging. Detection of target regions in the 3-D images enables in accurate description and sectional study of the regions [8]. Here for example, consider the head CT image of eight 2-D slices is subjected to 3-D segmentation using active contour models. In this process, mesh is designed for the head CT image based on which segmentation of the target region is performed. The mesh is formed with the help of the volumetric pixel values in all the x, y and z directions. The 2-D slice of the head CT image and mesh model designed for that 2-D slice of head CT image in all directions is defined in **Figure 2(a)** and **(b)** respectively. In **Figure 2(b)**, the axes of the mesh model describe the volumetric values (voxels) in all three directions representing the head CT image.

3-D segmentation of the image for every slices of the 2-D image is carried out through iterative applications of the active contour models. This segmentation process helps in segmenting the target region in all the slices. In this example, all the slices of head CT image undergo iterative contour segmentation for separation of the thoracic cavity [13]. In **Figure 3**, the iterative segmentation of each and every region of the thoracic cavity from the head CT image is shown. Segmentation of fine structures from the target object in an image is possible with these active contour models. Pham et al. describe the methods for medical image segmentation.

The application of active contour models for segmentation is used in various medical image processing techniques. 2-D and 3-D segmentation of the medical images is performed to obtain

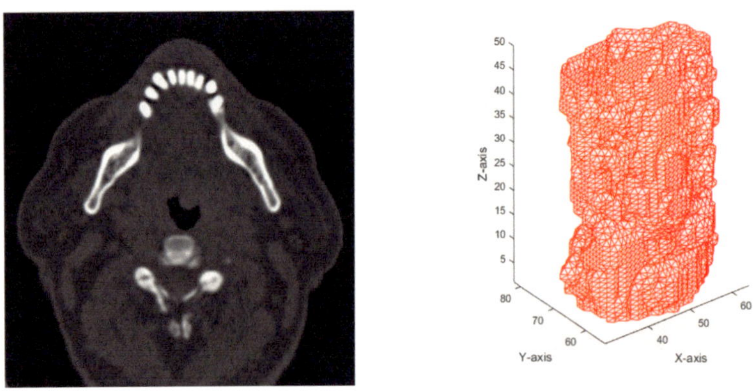

Figure 2. (a) 2-D slice of head CT image and (b) mesh model for the 2-D slice of head CT image.

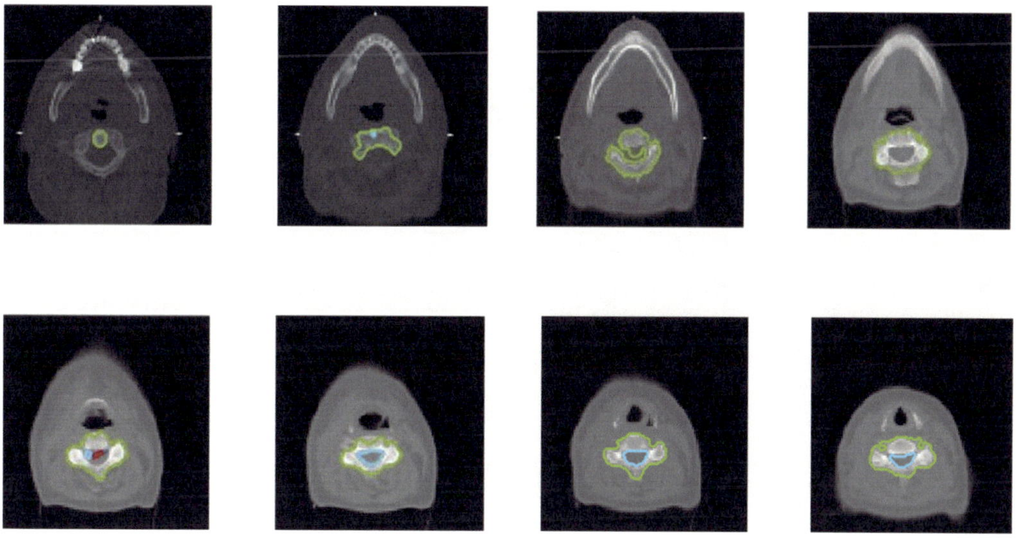

Figure 3. Iterative 3-D segmentation of head CT image using active contours.

the exact target object for identification, detection and diagnosis of any abnormal or unwanted changes in the human body. 2-D active contour models are used for segmentation of specific target area which possesses pixel information and in 3-D process of forming contour, the specific regions of voxel information are determined. Based on the information provided by the segmented region, further processing of the images occurs [16]. Active contour models are also used in 4-D segmentation such as motion tracking, stereo tracking of the movement of the internal regions [19].

Thus active contour models are used in various medical applications. The medical images from different modalities are considered for the description of active contour model and its types [28]. Active contour models used for medical image segmentation and processing are defined in this chapter. In the field of medicine, segmentation of target objects with accurate boundary lines is very much necessary for diagnosis and detection of any abnormalities in the body. This kind of segmentation is carried out with these models. In order to understand the application of active contour models in the field of medicine, these images are obtained from different authorised and standardised databases.Thus these medical images are considered to illustrate use of medical image processing. Traditional model and all the extended versions of the active contour models are described below in this chapter.

2.1. Snake model

Snake model is a technique that has the potential of solving wide class of segmentation cases. The model mainly works to identify and outlines the target object considered for segmentation. It uses a certain amount of prior knowledge about the target object contour especially for complex objects. Active snake model also called snakes generally configures by the application of spline focussed to minimise energy followed by various forces governing the image. Spline is a mathematical expression of a set of polynomials to derive geometric figures like curves. Spline of minimising energy guides the constraint forces and pulled with the help of internal and external image forces based on appropriate contour features. Snake model enacts deformable model to an image through energy minimisation. This model commonly uses cubic polynomial though higher order polynomials can be incorporated but usually avoided due to several undesirable local properties to confront with. Snake works efficiently with complex target objects by breaking down the figure into various smaller targets [1, 9].

Snake model is designed to vary its shape and position while tending to search through the minimal energy state. Snake propagates through the domain of the image to reduce the energy function, and intends to dynamically move to the local minimum. Snake is expressed by Eq. (1). The parametric form of the curve is exploited in the Snake model that has more advantages than utilising implicit and explicit curve forms

$$v(s,t) = \left(x\,(s,t), y(s,t)\right) \tag{1}$$

where x and y are the coordinates of the two-dimensional curve, v is spline parameter in the range 0–1, s is linear parameter ∈ [0,1] and t is time parameter ∈ [0, ∞].

The forces in snake include external forces as well as image forces that helps in feature identification. When the snake model moves around a closed curve, it moves with the influence of both internal and external energy to keep the total energy minimum. The total energy of active snake model is a summation of three types of energy namely (i) internal energy (E_i) which depends on the degree of the spline relating to the shape of the target image; (ii) external energy (E_e) which includes the external forces given by the user and also energy from various other factors; (iii) energy of the image under consideration (E_I) which conveys valuable data on the illumination of the spline representing the target object. The total energy defined for the contour formation in the snake model is given by Eq. (2).

$$E_T = E_i + E_e + E_I \tag{2}$$

$E_{internal}$ describes the internal energy which defines piecewise smoothness constraints in the contour, where α decides on how far the snake will be extended and the capacity of elasticity possible for the snake. β decides on the rigidity level for the snake. The internal energy is given by Eq. (3).

$$E_{internal} = \sigma\left|\frac{\partial v}{\partial s}\right|^2 + \beta\left|\frac{\partial^2 v}{\partial s^2}\right| \tag{3}$$

External energy constraints are mainly used to define the snake near the required local minimum. It may be described using high level interpretation and interaction.

$$E_{image} = w_1 I(x,y) + w_2\left|\nabla I(x,y)\right|^2 + \ldots, \tag{4}$$

The contour of the target object is shown in the above Eq. (4), where w_1 is called the line efficient and w_2 is called the edge efficient. According to the higher values of w_1 and w_2, snake will align itself to darker pixel regions in the case of positive value and it progresses towards the bright pixels when the value is negative. Snake model used for segmentation of various types of images.

The applications of active snake model are increasing in a tremendous manner especially in the various imaging fields. In medical imaging field, snake model is used segment one region of image which has special features compared to other regions of the image. Different applications of traditional snake model in medical imaging are optic disc and cup segmentation to detect glaucoma, cell image segmentation, vascular region and various other regions segmentation for diagnosis and study of disorders or abnormalities. For example, a slice of chest CT image is considered for segmentation using snake model. Chest CT image possesses the sections of internal organs like lungs and heart. In this image, snake model is applied for the segmentation of left lung from the chest image which is shown in **Figure 4**. Contour is developed around the left lung which can be used for further processing.

Boscolo et al. define the use of chest CT image for segmentation using traditional snake active contours. Specific region of segmentation is possible with these traditional active contour methods [26]. In the above example, specific lung region is separated from the image for extraction of features and diagnose the region whether it possesses any abnormalities or not in a computerised manner. The traditional method of active snake model has several inefficiencies like insensitivity to noises, false contour detection in high complex objects which are solved in advanced versions of contour methods.

2.2. Gradient vector flow model

Gradient vector flow model is an extended and well-defined technique of snake or active contour models. The traditional snake model possesses two limitations that is poor convergence performance of the contour for concave boundaries and when the snake curve flow is initiated at long distance from the minimum. Gradient vector flow model as an extension makes use of gradient vector flow field as energy constraint to define the contour flow.

Gradient vector flow (GVF) field is determined based on the following steps. The primary step is to detect the edge mapping function $f(x, y)$ from the image $I(x, y)$. Edge mapping function for binary images is described by Eq. (5), where $G_\sigma(x, y)$ is a 2D quassian function with the statistical parameter, standard deviation σ.

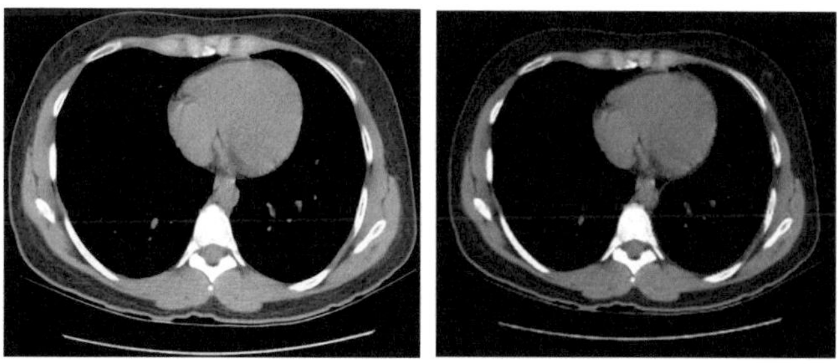

Figure 4. Segmentation of chest image using snake model.

$$f(x,y) = -G_\sigma(x,y)*I(x,y) \tag{5}$$

Edge map function for grey-scale images is given by Eq. (6) where the gradient operator is ∇

$$f(x,y) = -|\nabla[G_\sigma(x,y)*I(x,y)]|^2 \tag{6}$$

Gradient vector flow field is the equilibrium solution that reduces the functional energy. The functional energy possesses two different terms such as smoothing term and data term which depends on the parameter μ. The parameter value is based on the noise level in the image that is if the noise level is high then the parameter has to be increased. The main problem or limitation with gradient vector flow is the smoothing term that forms rounding of the edges of the contour. Therefore, increase in the value of μ reduces the rounding of edges but weakens the smoothing condition of the contour to a certain extent. The gradient vector flow is defined by the energy functional Eq. (7).

$$\varepsilon = \iint \mu\left(u_x{}^2 + v_x{}^2 + v_y{}^2\right) + |\nabla f|^2 |g - \nabla f|^2 \, dx\, dy \tag{7}$$

In this equation, g describes the gradient vector flow which can be derived based on the Euler equations. This equation defines the Laplacian operator that is defined by two different Eqs. (8) and (9).

$$\mu\nabla^2 u - (u - f_x)\left(f_x{}^2 + f_y{}^2\right) = 0 \tag{8}$$

$$\mu\nabla^2 v - (v - f_x)\left(f_x{}^2 + f_y{}^2\right) = 0 \tag{9}$$

Computational solutions to calculate f_x and f_y in the equation are obtained by using common gradient operators such as sobel, prewitt, or isotropic operators. Based on these parameters the gradient vector flow field is defined. After the determination of GVF field g(x,y) it is used to replace the energy constraints in the traditional snake model. With these constraints, the continuous computation of the curve flow occurs iteratively for structural defining of the contour [4].

Gradient vector flow model can be used in all higher dimensions based on the minimum of the energy function. In two-dimensional image regions, a time variable t is introduced for solving the Euler equations. The Euler equation can be used to define entire target object as a deformable contour through iteration towards a steady state value. Thus the equations obtained are used instead of the external force in the traditional snake model. Contour of the target object from the image is defined based on the edge mapping function and gradient vector flow field. The gradient vector flow model is used for the segmentation of exact target region compared to the snake model.

The gradient vector flow model is an extended version of snake model used in various image processing applications especially in medical image processing. In medical imaging, the segmentation of regions with specific parameters is carried out with the help of active contour models. Because these models develop a contour around the target object and segregates it from the image. The segmented image possesses only the required information of the target object [10].

For example, the breast mammogram obtained from a standard database undergoes gradient vector flow active contour model. This model defines the boundaries of the breast region and regions of calcification in the mammogram image section. The segmentation of breast mammogram with the highlighted calcification regions is shown in **Figure 5**. In the mammogram image segmentation, the calcified regions are highlighted with the gradient vector flow contours which help in computerised early diagnosis and detection of calcification in breast regions. Ferrari et al. describes the segmentation of boundaries of the calcified region in breast mammogram [27]. Gradient vector flow field also uses the minimum energy function for segmentation of cardiac and brain regions. This model helps in motion tracking of the various regions in the human body especially pumping action of the heart and muscular activities of various regions.

Gradient vector flow model is used for all types of images obtained from different imaging modalities. Thus extended version of snake in the form of gradient vector field is used in all medical image processing applications.

2.3. Balloon model

A snake model is not attracted to distant edges. The snake model will shrink inner side, if no substantial images forces are acting upon it. A snake larger than the minima contour will eventually shrink into it, but a snake smaller than minima contour will not find the minima and instead continue to shrink. In order to overcome the limitations of snake model, balloon model was introduced in which inflation term is induced into the forces acting on the snake [3]. The inflation force can overpower forces from weak edges, amplifying the issue with localisation of initial guess. The additional inflation force is given by Eq. (10) with $\vec{n}(s)$ as normal unity vector of the curve and k_1 as magnitude of the curve.

$$F_{inflation} = k_1 \vec{n}(s) \tag{10}$$

Here k_1 should possess similar magnitude as that of the image normalisation vector k and must have smaller value that allows the forces in the image edges to adjust with the inflation force given additional to the internal and external energy.

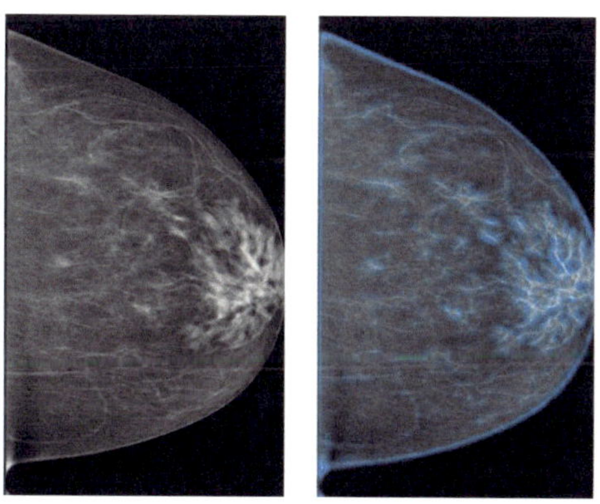

Figure 5. Breast mammogram segmentation using gradient vector flow (GVF) model.

An overview of this algorithm, it will locate an area in the volume, then place a icosahedron in that area such that it contains no points. Expand (or) subdivide the icosahedron so that it approximates the volume. Thus the algorithm starts with a small icosahedron inside the object. Each vertex is connected to its neighbours by springs that inflate each triangle or segment along the normal based on inflation pressure inside the sphere. With respect to depth, start with range images where the images are joined to a single point cloud. Manually insert the starting point of icosahedron hence, if it is difficult to compute do it by hand. Then place the icosahedron in a fixed location to develop a contour.

The major two forces act on each vertex. Inflation force is used to push the vertices out and spring force is calculated based upon one ring neighbourhood of each vertex. Inflation force is calculated based upon normality of value of points in the contour. Expansion algorithm is a set of instructions used to create a front of the icosahedron which has all the faces. At first, insert the front section into the instructions queue. For each vertex in the front, it is used to calculate the spring force and inflation force. Now, compute the new location. Compute nearest point from the dataset. Then, update the co-ordinator. Later, discard the anchored triangles in the region of interest. The expanding triangles will reconstruct the surface less accurately due to their large size. While expanding the spring forces between vertices become very large. Subdivide triangles to reduce force. Triangles are subdivided so that no T shaped junctions exist in forming the contour. Long and skinny triangles are reconnected to be wide and short. A triangle becomes anchored once it reaches the surface of the point cloud. This is determined by testing for intersection with the point set based on vertex normal. Once a triangle is anchored it has no longer moves, all the vertices are stationary [13].

Three issues arise from using the balloon model. Instead of shrinking, the snake expands into the minima and will not find minima contour smaller than it. The outward force causes the contour to be slightly larger than the actual minima. This can be solved by decreasing the balloon force after a solution has been found. Computation is done by performing the intersection of a ray with a range image. Iterative process requires refinement of approximation. All range scans have to be looked to get a result. Holes are handled similarly to anchoring process. Noise is broken into two categories namely misalignment of range scans, scan errors mostly outliers. Both these areas are handled by intersection algorithm and filtering.

Balloon model is used in the segmentation of different medical images. The application is mainly used for presenting a novel model for segmenting 2-D image and reconstructing 3-D meshes which guarantees a waterlight mesh. In 2-D segmentation, the contour separates the region of pixels with specific feature. Contour is formed for separation of lesions, tissue regions, infected cells, and parasites from the images. 3-D mesh formation is mainly used in the reconstruction of 3-D images from different imaging modalities [10]. 3-D models can also be designed for artificial implants using mesh technique based on the inflation balloon force.

One of the examples for 2-D segmentation of images using balloon model is skin lesion segmentation. The segmentation of lesion from the dermal image is shown in **Figure 6**. In general, skin lesion segmentation from the dermal images is very much necessary for the early detection of skin cancer which is becoming predominant in all tropical countries. Thus balloon model is commonly used for segmentation of lesions because the inflation force defines an

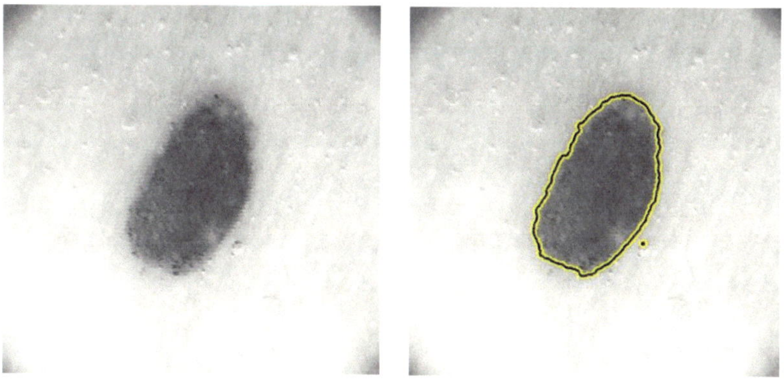

Figure 6. Skin lesion segregation from the dermal images using balloon models.

accurate contour [31, 32]. These contours are used for further processing and prediction of skin cancer. The main disadvantage of the balloon model is slow processing that it is difficult to handle sharp edges and it has a manual object placement. Balloon model is widely used in analysing the extraction of specific image contour.

2.4. Geometric or geodesic active contour models

Geometric active contour or geodesic active contour (GAC) is a type of contour models that modifies the smooth curve defined in the Euclidean plan by moving the points of the curve perpendicular. The motion of the points is at a speed proportional to the curvature of the region in the image. Contours are described based on the geometric flow of curve and detection of objects in the image. Geometric flow includes both internal and external measures of geometry in the region of interest. Geometric alternative for snakes is used in the process of detection of objects in an image. These contour models largely depend on the level set functions that describe the specific regions in the image for segmentation [5, 6].

Geometric contours define a initial curve C_0 with the flow of geometry given by the planar contour evolution Eq. (11) with g as the edge indicator scalar function, $k\vec{N}$ as curvature vector, $\vec{N}$ as normal vector to the curve and v as arbitrary constant.

$$C_t = g(C)(k - v)\,\vec{N} \tag{11}$$

The curve evolution continues to propagate until the g value becomes zero that indicates the curve reaches edge of the region or object required from the image. In this method of contour model, snake parameter is replaced by Euclidean arc length which is defined as given in Eq. (12)

$$ds = |Cp|\,dp \tag{12}$$

Euclidean arc length describes the irregular length of the curve based on the curvature and the energy forces. Internal and external energy forces are coupled together which leads to minimum of the functional derivative of geometric curve flow. Differential evolution of curvature of the region in an image is given by the Euler Lagrange Eq. (13) in which C is defined as signed distance function [20].

$$\frac{dC}{dt} = \left(g(C)k - \left\langle \nabla g, \vec{N} \right\rangle\right) \vec{N} \tag{13}$$

Geometric active contour depends on the level set function and geometric planar curve evolution which describes the region for segmentation. By adding an area of minimising region (balloon force), propagation of contour occurs internal by minimisation of the interior energy. Therefore, Euler Lagrange equation is determined as the deepest descent and is given by Eq. (14).

$$\frac{dC}{dt} = \left(g(C)k - \left\langle \nabla g, \vec{N} \right\rangle - \sigma g(C)\right) \vec{N} \tag{14}$$

Contour models use the energy forces for geometric flow curve description. Geometric contours can be obtained based on regions and edges in the curvature of the image [12].

Edge-based geometric active contours define a geometric flow curve evolution depending on the gradients of edges or boundaries in the image that undergoes contour segmentation. Edge-based geometric models possess fast computation speed and can simultaneously segment different regions of different intensities. In some regions, penetration of gap in-between the curvature occurs due to large gradient magnitudes. These geometric models are sensitive to local maximum gradient computation which is used in defining the contours. These limitations can be fixed by increasing the curvature weight and advection weight respectively.

Region-based geometric contour models are based on either the variance inside and outside contour or the squared difference between average intensities inside and outside the contours along with the total contour length. This type of contour model supports different image properties not only edges which may include texture and other geometrical features. In these contours, computation of multiple groups or segments is not possible but less sensitive to noise [15].

Geometric active contours are mainly employed in medical image computing especially in image-based segmentation. In this, image from any imaging modality is considered for segmentation, to study, process and analyse the regions of interest. These regions may be described as any abnormality formed in the internal regions or organs of the human body like blood clots, injuries, lesions, cell abnormality, metabolic interruptions, biomolecule disruptions and so on. Metabolic changes in the regions or organs can be studied with the help of geodesic contours. Geodesic or geometric contours are mainly based on the geometric measures, and curvature flow based on segmentation process occurs. In this example, fundus image of the eye is segmented with the geometric measures that describes the curvature of the eye ball, optic disc localisation and path of the fine nerve endings. Fundus image mainly contributes to the curvature and position of the optic disc.

In this, geometric flow defines the curvature of eye ball, so abnormalities based on curvature can be obtained. Stąpor et al. define the fundus eye image segmentation with different techniques. One among them is geodesic active contour model [30]. Optic disc localisation is performed with the mapping level set functions. The optic disc is segmented as an elevated structure possessing the fine retinal vessels and nerve endings [34]. Contour of each and every fine structure in the image is described through geometric or geodesic active contours [7, 29]. This property of the active contour model can be used more effectively in 3-D image construction and mapping. In **Figure 7**, segmentation of fundus image for optic disc localisation is shown.

Recent applications of geometric or geodesic active contours include 3-D medical image segmentation and 3-D motion tracking and segmentation of moving objects in medical imaging. Segmentation of medical images using geometric or geodesic active contour models has increased largely for accurate separation or segregation of required regions. Thus fine and absolute details of the medical images can be obtained and even three-dimensional data can be derived using this geodesic contour model.

In general, active contour models possess different extended versions with change either in the form of energy constraints or forces. New contour models are designed for the segmentation of absolute details of the image. One of the active contour models in which the constraints and energy forces are used to develop a contour around the edges of the target object. In order to study the membrane structures, edge-based contour models are used. Region-based active contour models are developed for 3-D segmentation of images. These contour models develop contour boundaries with energy forces required for the particular region of interest [23].

Fuzzy energy-based active contour models are designed for segmentation process in which fuzzy logic is applied by changing the localised membership values for each iteration. These contour models are used for multiple object segmentation [21]. 3-D adaptive crisp active contour model is a newly developed technique for 3-D segmentation of medical images especially used for CT lung image segmentation. Adaptive energy constraints are used for automatic initialisation of deformable contours [24]. Other extended version of active contour model is designed based on the local and global details of intensity in an image. The statistical numerical and level set function determines the intensity inside and outside the contour of the image. With less iteration, these contour models can be used for medical image segmentation [25, 34].

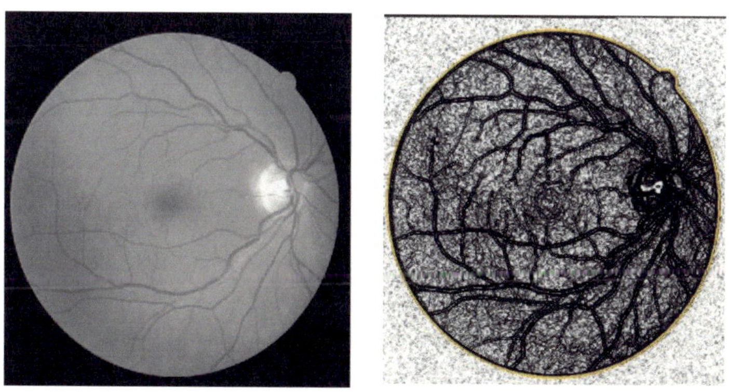

Figure 7. Fundus image segmentation using geodesic active contours.

Frequency-tuned active contour model uses predefined frequency filters to describe the process of segmentation. Gaussian difference is used to remove high range of noise and intensity variations which are obtained using region-based active contour models. This contour model allows selective segmentation and can effectively segment the near texture regions in an image. The contour models are very useful in processing various image datasets and especially for segmentation of real-time optical coherence tomography images [22]. Thus there are different types of extended active contour models used in various image processing applications.

Active contour models of various different forms are defined in this chapter to illustrate the process of target image segmentation. These models are mainly used to form a deformable contour around the target objects more effectively. Energy forces describe a specific contour for the required region based on various features. This type of image segmentation technique is used in different applications. Especially in the field of medical imaging, segmentation of particular regions is very necessary for diagnosis and detection of abnormalities. Active contour models are best suitable for target object segmentation.

3. Conclusions

Segmentation is a technique to describe, define and segregate regions of interest. Image segmentation is a process mainly to derive the region, curvature or contour of the required targeted region from the image. Segmentation in an image depends on various features and parameters. Active contour models are defined for image segmentation based on the curve flow, curvature and contour to obtain the exact target region or segment in the image for future analysis and processing. Contour models are used in processing various images from different modalities. Active contours segregate the regions of required pixel intensities based on the energy forces and conditions. Different types of active contour models are used in the process of segmentation.

In this chapter, active contour models used for the image segmentation process is described in detail. The different types of active contour models defined are traditional snake, balloon, gradient vector flow and geodesic active contour model. In which snake model depends on the internal and external forces exerted by the contour curve. Balloon model similar to snakes uses an additional inflation force to define the curvature. In gradient vector flow model, the contour is described based on the gradient vectors of the curve flow. Geometric model defines the contour using the geometric flow curve and energy forces.

Active contour models are applied in different fields for image segmentation process. In medical imaging field, segmentation of images from different regions of the human body is carried out to study, analyse, diagnose and detect abnormalities. Lesions, blood clotting, abnormal outgrowths, cysts, tumours, cancer cells, small aneurysms, inflations and various other diverse abnormalities can be segmented from the medical images for easily analysis and diagnosis [18]. The application of each and every active contour model described in this chapter is related to medical image processing. Medical images from different modalities are considered for the description of the contour models.

3-D segmentation of the contours defined in the target region can be used for further construction and analysis of 3-D images [33]. Active contour models are also useful for mesh formations. These formations help in designing 3-D structures and models. 2-D segmentation of active contour models is more elaborately described in this chapter of image segmentation process. Each active contour model is illustrated with an example describing the segmentation process and algorithms in the field of medical imaging. Different medical images are defined in the examples to provide a clear understanding about the active contour models. Active contour models of different types are used for image segmentation in the various field but widely used in medicine for the early diagnosis and detection of abnormalities in a computerised manner. Thus automatic segmentation of the medical images for diagnosis and study is performed with the active contour models.

Author details

R.J. Hemalatha*, T.R. Thamizhvani, A. Josephin Arockia Dhivya, Josline Elsa Joseph, Bincy Babu and R. Chandrasekaran

*Address all correspondence to: rjhemalatha@gmail.com

Department of Biomedical Engineering, Vels Institute of Science, Technology and Advanced Studies (Deemed to be University), Chennai, India

References

[1] Kass M, Witkin A, Terzopoulos D. Snakes: Active contour models. International Journal of Computer Vision. 1988;**1**:321-331. DOI: 10.1007/BF00133570

[2] Chan TF, Vese LA. Active contours without edges. IEEE Transactions on Image Processing. 2001;**10**:266-277. DOI: 10.1109/83.902291

[3] Laurent Cohen D. On active contour models and balloons. CVGIP: Image Understanding. 2004;**53**:211-218. DOI: 10.1016/1049-9660(91)90028-N

[4] Xu C, Prince JL. Gradient vector flow: A new external force for snakes. In: Proceedings of the IEEE Conference on Computer Vision and Pattern Recognition (CVPR '97); 17–19 June 1997; Puerto Rico, USA: IEEE; 1991. pp. 66-71

[5] Goldenberg R, Kimmel R, Rivlin E, Rudzsky M. Fast geodesic active contours. IEEE Transactions on Image Processing. 2001;**10**:1467-1475. DOI: 10.1109/83.951533

[6] Caselles V, Kimmel R, Sapiro G. Geodesic active contours. International Journal of Computer Vision. 1997;**22**:61-79. DOI: 10.1023/A:1007979827043.

[7] Agarwal A, Issac A, Singh A, Dutta MK. Automatic imaging method for optic disc segmentation using morphological techniques and active contour fitting. In: Proceedings

of the Ninth International Conference on Contemporary Computing (IC3); 11–13 August 2016; Noida, India: IEEE; 2017. pp. 1-5

[8] Saha R, Bhowmik MK. Active contour models for medical applications. In: Mandal JK, Mukhopadhyay S, Pal T, editors. Handbook of Research on Natural Computing for Optimization Problems. 2nd ed. Dauphin County, Pennsylvania: IGI Global; 2016. pp. 937-959. DOI: 10.4018/978-1-5225-0058-2.ch038

[9] Li C, Kao C-Y, Gore JC, Ding Z. Implicit active contours driven by local binary fitting energy. In: Proceedings of the IEEE Conference on Computer Vision and Pattern Recognition (CVPR '07); 17–22 June 2007; Minneapolis, USA: IEEE; 2007. pp. 1-7

[10] Khadidos A, Sanchez V, Li C-T. Active contours based on weighted gradient vector flow and balloon forces for medical image segmentation. In: Proceedings of the IEEE International Conference on Image Processing (ICIP); 27–30 October 2014; Paris, France: IEEE; 2014. pp. 902-906

[11] Suetens P, Bellon E, Vandermeulen D, Smet M, Marchal G, Nuyts J, Mortelmans L. Image segmentation: Methods and applications in diagnostic radiology and nuclear medicine. European Journal of Radiology. 1993;**17**:14-21. DOI: 10.1016/0720-048X(93)90023-G

[12] Caselles V, Catté F, Coll T, Dibos F. A geometric model for active contours in image processing. Numerische Mathematik. 1993;**66**:1-31. DOI: 10.1007/BF01385685

[13] Cohen LD, Cohen I. Finite-element methods for active contour models and balloons for 2-D and 3-D images. IEEE Transactions on Pattern Analysis and Machine Intelligence. 1993;**15**:1131-1147. DOI: 10.1109/34.244675

[14] Eviatar H, Somorjai RL. A fast, simple active contour algorithm for biomedical images. Pattern Recognition Letters. 1996;**17**:969-974. DOI: 10.1016/0167-8655(96)00054-2

[15] Lankton S, Tannenbaum A. Localizing region-based active contours. IEEE Transactions on Image Processing. 2008;**17**:2029-2039. DOI: 10.1109/TIP.2008.2004611

[16] Davatzikos CA, Prince JL. An active contour model for mapping the cortex. IEEE Transactions on Medical Imaging. 1995;**14**:65-80. DOI: 10.1109/42.370403

[17] Michailovich O, Rathi Y, Tannenbaum A. Image segmentation using active contours driven by Bhattacharyya gradient flow. IEEE Transactions on Image Processing. 2007;**16**: 2787-2801. DOI: 10.1109/TIP.2007.908073

[18] Mclnerney T, Terzopoulos D. Deformable models in medical image analysis: A survey. Medical Image Analysis. 1996;**1**:91-108. DOI: 10.1016/S1361-8415(96)80007-7

[19] Mikic I, Krucinski S, Thomas JD. Segmentation and tracking in echocardiographic sequences: Active contours guided by optical flow estimates. IEEE Transactions on Medical Imaging. 1998;**17**:274-284. DOI: 10.1109/42.700739

[20] Chen Y, Tagare HD, Thiruvenkadam S, Huang F, Wilson D, Gopinath KS, Briggs RW, Geiser EA. Using prior shapes in geometric active contours in a variational framework. International Journal of Computer Vision. 2002;**50**:315-328. DOI: 10.1023/A:1020878408985

[21] Shi J, Wu J, Anisetti M, Damiani E, Jeon G. An interval type-2 fuzzy active contour model for auroral oval segmentation. Soft Computing. 2017;**21**:2325-2345. DOI: 10.1007/s00500-015-1943-7

[22] Guo Q, Sun S, Ren X, Dong F, Gao BZ, Feng W. Frequency tuned active contour model. Neurocomputing. 2018;**275**:2307-2316. DOI: 10.1016/j.neucom.2017.11.003

[23] Liu C, Xiao Y, Yang J. A coastline detection method in polarimetric SAR images mixing the region-based and edge-based active contour models. IEEE Transactions on Geoscience and Remote Sensing. 2017;**55**:3735-3747. DOI: 10.1109/TGRS.2017.2679112

[24] Filho PPR, Cortez PC, da Silva Barros AC, Albuquerque VHC, Tavares JMRS. Novel and powerful 3D adaptive crisp active contour method applied in the segmentation of CT lung images. Medical Image Analysis. 2017;**35**:503-516. DOI: 10.1016/j.media.2016.09.002

[25] Niu S, Chen Q, de Sisternes L, Ji Z, Zhou Z, Rubin DL. Robust noise region-based active contour model via local similarity factor for image segmentation. Pattern Recognition. 2017;**61**:104-119. DOI: 10.106/j.patcog.2016.07.022

[26] Boscolo R, Brown MS, McNitt-Gray MF. Medical image segmentation with knowledge-guided robust active contours. Radiographics. 2002;**22**:437-446. DOI: 10.1148/radiographics.22.2.g02mr26437

[27] Ferrari RJ, Frere AF, Rangayyan RM, Desautels JEL, Borges RA. Identification of the breast boundary in mammograms using active contour models. Medical and Biological Engineering and Computing. 2004;**42**:201-208. DOI: 10.1007/BF02344632

[28] Pham DL, Xu C, Prince JL. Current methods in medical image segmentation. Annual Review of Biomedical Engineering. 2000;**2**:315-337. DOI: 10.1146/annurev.bioeng.2.1.315

[29] Malek J, Abdallah MB, Mansour A, Tourki R. Automated optic disc detection in retinal images by applying region-based active contour model in a variational level set formulation. In: Proceedings of International Conference on Computer Vision in Remote Sensing (CVRS); 16–18 December 2012; Xiamen, China: IEEE; 2013. pp. 117-121

[30] Stąpor K, Świtonski A, Chrastek R, Michelson G. Segmentation of fundus eye images using methods of mathematical morphology for glaucoma diagnosis. In: Proceedings of International Conference on Computational Science (ICCS); 6–9 June 2004; Krakow, Poland: Springer; 2004. pp. 41-48

[31] Emre Celebi M, Lyatomi H, Schaefer G, Stoecker WV. Lesion border detection in dermoscopy images. Computerized Medical Imaging and Graphics. 2009;**33**:148-153. DOI: 10.1016/j.compmedimag.2008.11.002

[32] Erkol B, Moss RH, Joe Stanley R, Stoecker WV, Hvatum E. Automatic lesion boundary detection in dermoscopy images using gradient vector flow snakes. Skin Research and Technology. 2005;**11**:17-26. DOI: 10.1111/j.1600-0846.2005.00092.x

[33] Yushkevich PA, Piven J, Hazlett HC, Smith RG, Ho S, Gee JC, Gerig G. User-guided 3D active contour segmentation of anatomical structures: Significantly improved efficiency and reliability. NeuroImage. 2006;**31**:1116-1128. DOI: 10.1016/j.neuroimage.2006.01.015

[34] Al-Diri B, Hunter A, Steel D. An active contour model for segmenting and measuring retinal vessels. IEEE Transactions on Medical Imaging. 2009;**28**:1488-1497. DOI: 10.1109/TMI.2009.2017941

Section 2

Image Analysis Examples

Chapter 3

Medical and Biological Image Analysis

Abdelkader Moumen

Additional information is available at the end of the chapter

http://dx.doi.org/10.5772/intechopen.75491

Abstract

Today, technology and information communication are deeply embedded in our life. Information is present and used in many forms: electronic documents, audio, videos, photos, etc. Recent advances in technology, particularly in the computer industry and communication, have motivated organisations to replace their traditional manually stored and exchanged records with computer systems and digital documents for secure storage and smooth transmission. Medical and biological image processing is a numerical method and technique for modifying a digital image to improve or extract information. The main stages of image processing are:

1. **acquisition of the image:** by cameras, radars, sensors and so on;

2. **image enhancement:** Highlight some components of the image or reveal details and make the image clear.

3. **image restoration:** can be considered as inverting the dosages caused by a processor software. We rely on mathematical or probabilistic models for the degradation of an image; and

4. **image segmentation:** dividing the image into distinct elements or partitioning the image into objects. In this chapter, we discuss the medical and biological image and related topics such as classification of security of these data, the problem of security.

Keywords: digital image, medical image, biological image, encryption, decryption, evaluation parameters

1. Introduction

With the rapid development of multimedia technologies and communication networks and the evolution of equipment that is capable of acquiring, archiving and to transmit images and videos at reasonable costs, which favours their use in several areas such as computer vision, medical imaging, multimedia systems, satellite imagery, telemedicine, and so on. These data are exchanged via channels that are not always secure, most of them are transmitted over open networks, much of this information is confidential or private. Indeed, this data can be easily intercepted or modified by attackers or by unauthorised users. The security of this information during transfer or storage has become more important and has attracted a lot of attention.

The use of medical imaging and biological image by professionals has remarkably evolved in recent years due to the development of digital technologies. It allows an increasingly in-depth investigation of organs through more efficient radiology systems. The statistical approach induced by the use of computer tools induces treatments on images in very high definition, so a modality like a scanner produces images of the size of the order of 10 MB and a complete examination reaches 500 MB. This critical volume not only posed the problem of the storage, circulation and exchange of this digital information between professionals, but also raised security problems.

2. Digital image

Long before the invention of the computer, the man had chosen a simple way of communication that does not require any specialised knowledge except that of to draw, this method is to draw and design images. First of all, let us agree on the term 'image', the definition of model in the dictionary: [A representation of the external form of a person or thing in art]. For a computer, the display support of a digital image is the screen.

The development of communication media and storage media has dramatically transformed the means of communication. New technologies are mostly based on the exchange and storage of multimedia data and especially digital images. As a result, the digital image becomes plenty. Moreover, it is indispensable in several fields, notably communication [1]. In this section, we study the major categories of images and medical image and biological image. Also, we present the most well-known evaluation parameters of encrypted images.

A colour digital image is a computer file, which can be opened with an image viewing program. Once the image is open in real size, it is in the form of a rectangle consisting of a set of coloured points. A digital image is saved as a file. It is characterised by three elements:

1. Its type and format.
2. Its resolution in pixels.
3. Its colour depth.

2.1. The matrix image

This type of images are prevalent and the most widespread, a digital image matrix, also called the BITMAP image, can be considered as a matrix or an ordered set of two- or three-dimensional digital data.

http://dx.doi.org/10.5772/intechopen.75491

The row and column indices identify the points in the image. The elements of the matrix are the elementary units of the image, they are called pixels or picture elements; the pixel is an abbreviation for PICture ELement [1, 2]. The number of rows of this matrix is m, and n represents the number of columns, and the product m × n gives us the size of the image. The resolution of an image is defined by the number of pixels per unit length. Therefore, we can build an image 2D as an array of values in which a position is matched on a plane (x, y) and a colour to visualise the image on an electronic medium.

It is simply a grid of thousands of pixels representing the successive colour points of the image. Each pixel is a very small square having precise coordinates and precise colour, in this way, the image then becomes a grid of pixels. This is the technique used in medical and biological image capture devices and digital cameras or scanners. Bitmap images are fully adapted to the world of photography. On the other hand, the more the quality of the image, the more voluminous is the file. Most popular formats are JPEG, PNG and GIF.

2.2. The vector image

It is a digital image composed of geometric objects and created from mathematical equations (such as a circle, an arc, a curve, a straight line, a polygon) and parameters (like position, dimensions, colour). Each object is defined mathematically by equations and attributes like the position, colour, and so on. For example, the vector image of a circle is defined by type attributes such as centre position, radius and a straight line drawn between the points (x 1, y 1) and (x 2, y 2). We cannot present all the images in a vectorial way, and this is mainly the case of realistic photos that are matrix images. A vector image cannot be displayed directly on a screen. It must be transformed into a matrix type image.

These images are mainly used to make diagrams or plans in industrial software such as Desktop Publishing (PAO), CAD (Computer Aided Drawing), AutoCAD, CATIA, Illustrator and the tools of 3D design (like 3DSMax, Maya). The best-known formats are EPS, EMF and Windows Metafile (WMF).

Unlike matrix images, in the vector image, the positions and colours of the objects are not fixed, and they are calculated dynamically by the viewing software. In other words, to display a line, for example, the software determines the starting point, the point of arrival and the trajectory to follow. Then, it calculates and positions all the pixels necessary to display this line. The same procedure can be used for more complex shapes and colours.

Vector images are rather light, that is, small file size. Also, because they consist only of mathematical entities, they have the famous property of being able to be enlarged without limit, each line and each form being dynamically recalculated (**Figures 1(a), (b)** and **2(a), (b)**). On the other hand, they are rather dedicated to creating relatively simple renderings such as diagrams, etc.

Difficult indeed to create such renderings of landscapes, details, games of shadows with vector image that does not allow realism.

In **Figure 1**, we see that when we make a zoom on matrix image, the quality and the clarity of the zoomed image will be decreased. On the other hand, in **Figure 2**, when we zoom a vector image, the zoomed image does not lose the quality.

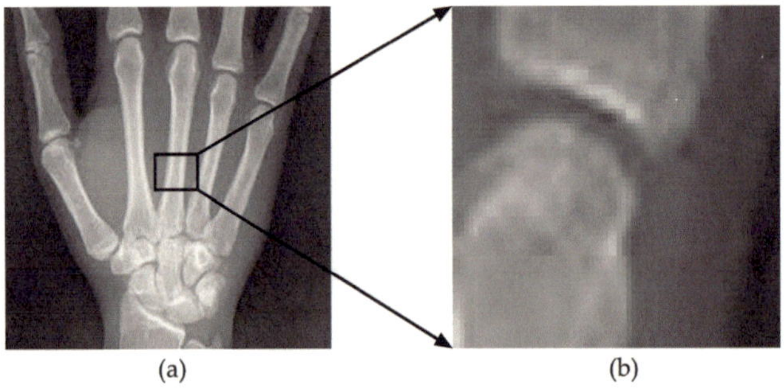

Figure 1. Zoom on matrix image: decrease of the quality of the image.

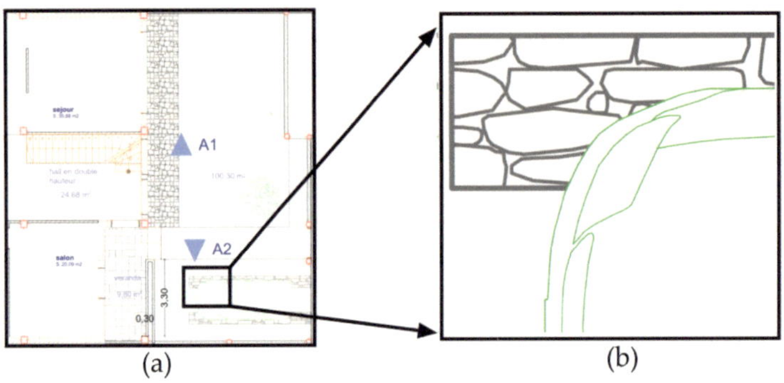

Figure 2. Zoom on vector image: does not lose the quality of the image.

3. Medical and biological image

Medical and biological imaging is a set of techniques consisting of imaging the different regions of the body. The use of the medical and biological images allows a deeper and deeper investigation of organs through radiology, and it is also used in biomedical research to understand better how the body works.

The beginning medical imaging is the result of the work of Wilhelm Röntgen on the X-rays in 1895, and he made the first anatomical X-ray images of his wife Anna Berthe Roentgen. He received the Nobel Prize in Physics in 1901. There exist several types of medical and biological imaging that are more or less adapted according to the area of study. We distinguish in particular [3, 4]:

1. **Images of gamma rays:** the biological body is injected with radioactive isotopes that emit gamma rays, and the emissions are collected with detectors to produce an image.
2. **Radiology, which uses X-rays:** X-rays are one of the oldest sources of electromagnetic radiation used in medical and biological imaging. It is used for diagnostics and also in industry and astronomy.

3. **Magnetic resonance imaging (MRI):** it is a powerful medical diagnostic technique that provides three-dimensional images in an anatomically accurate cut. These examinations use ultrasound, sound waves at very high frequencies (above 20,000 Hz). MRI is based on the physical phenomenon of nuclear magnetic resonance. It is simply a question of observing the nuclear magnetic resonance of the protons of the water contained in the organism.

Medical and biological images are real images, they cannot be calculated; therefore, they are matrix images. The evolution of multimedia and communication technologies has consequences in the field of health through the provision of new means of sharing and remote access like picture archiving communication systems (PACS) and the adoption of new standards. The need for a measure appeared after the development of the media digital and image networks. The medical community has actively set standards for digitally exchanging patient records and in particular, medical images, among the objectives of these criteria, to make the software solutions more efficient. A standard of medical information exchange is a convention between professionals to access and exchange and secure the data. Among the criteria existing on the market, it is possible to quote [4, 5]:

1. Digital Imaging and Communication in Medicine (DICOM):

   Digital Imaging and Communication in Medicine (DICOM) is the global standard for the management of medical images and their environment, and it was created in 1985 by the American College of Radiology (ACR) and the National Electric Manufacturers Association (NEMA) to standardise the data transmitted between different radiology devices [6]. This standard not only defines a file format but also a data transmission protocol. The DICOM standard is now used by most manufacturers of medical imaging equipment.

2. Integrating the Healthcare Enterprise:

   Integrating the Healthcare Enterprise (IHE) is an initiative of health professionals to ensure better interoperability between systems [7]. It proposes the use of standards for the exchange of clinical and administrative information such as DICOM for the image and health level 7 (HL7) for messages between medical software.

3. Hospital Information Systems:

   Hospital Information Systems (SIH) is an information system applied to health facilities such as hospitals, clinics, radiology centres, analysis centres and medical offices? It covers all the systems of functioning in a health facility such as administrative system, accounting system, logistics and stock system, medical informatics, and so on.

4. Radiological Information Systems:

   Information system is usually computer-assisted, designed to store, manipulate and search for information. It manages the planning and management of certain administrative and clinical activities such as patient identification and follow-up, appointment management, the realisation of the exams, dictation of the report, invoicing, and so on.

5. Health Level 7:

Health Level 7 (HL7) is a standard that defines a format for exchanged clinical electronic data [8]. This information can be financials or administrative.

3.1. Colour coding

For a digital image, we can distinguish three main types of colours [1] (**Figure 3**):

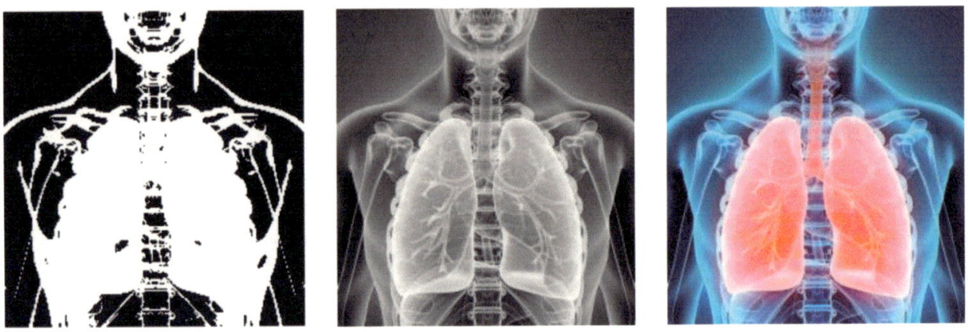

(a) (b) (c)

Figure 3. (a) Binary image, (b) greyscale image and (c) colour image.

3.1.1. Binary images

Binary images are pixel matrices where the content of each element can only take values 0 for black or 1 for the white colour (**Figure 3(a)**). Therefore, the number of colours is only of two, and the rendering of the image is sometimes sufficient in some cases.

The first applications adapted well to this type of images. In the beginnings of digital image processing, we have the problem of calculation time and memory space. Therefore, it did not allow processing of complex images. Binary images are a simple context allowing formalisation of mathematical problems by tools such as topology. Also, in the field of industrial vision such as fault detection, quality control, measurement, and so on, we often consider the binary image as a mandatory step, generally following the phase of segmentation, hence the importance of this type of images.

3.1.2. Grayscale images

Greyscale images are coded on 8 bits (corresponding to 1 byte), and in this case, we get $2^{24} = 256$ intensities between 0 and 255 which represents, respectively, black and white (**Figure 3(b)**). It is an image that offers several levels of intensity ranging from black to white. Greyscale coding offers more shades than simple black and white. A total of 255 different grey levels are sufficient for the presentation of most medical and biological objects, the advantage of greyscale images is it occupies less space, and the treatment is fluid.

3.1.3. Colour images

In this coding, the image is broken down in general into three planes: red, green and blue (**Figure 3(c)**). The colour of a pixel is obtained, as the painter would mix the basic colours. Each pixel is represented by a vector consisting of red, green and blue components.

We describe one of the most commonly used principles. RGB coding: The principle consists of mixing the three colours: red, green and blue (denoted RGB) (see **Table 1**). With these three colours, we obtain a whole palette of shades ranging from black to white. Each colour is associated with 1 byte (256 levels of brightness) of each of the fundamental colours.

Red	Green	Blue	Colour
0	0	0	Black
255	0	0	Red
0	255	0	Green
0	0	255	Blue
128	128	128	Grey
255	255	255	White

Table 1. Principle of RGB colour coding.

A 'colour' pixel is then coded with 3 (or 24-bit) bytes, and then, it is possible to obtain colour possibilities, that is, 16 million different colours (16,777,216 = 2^{24}).

There are other types of encoding colours, and the best known are TSL, CMY, CIE, YUV, and YIQ.

4. Evaluation methods

Any image processing changes the pixels relative to the original image. A robust ciphering algorithm must make these changes irregularly and at the same time, maximise the difference between the pixel values of the original image and the ciphered image. The encrypted image must be independent of the original image, and the final image must not reveal the characteristics of the plaintext image.

One of the oldest and best-known measures is visual inspection; with the advancement of cryptanalysis techniques, the visual inspection is no longer sufficient to examine the power of a ciphering algorithm. Therefore, the use of quantitative factors is necessary to judge a cryptosystem [9] better.

Factors that measure the quality of the recording techniques can be classified into two families [4, 10]:

1. **Correlation:** This family measures the ability of the algorithm to have a weak relationship between the original image and the encrypted image. In this way, five measures are studied: the histogram, the correlation coefficient, entropy, irregular gap and noise resistance.

2. **Diffusion:** This second family evaluates the characteristics of diffusion of the algorithm. In this family, two measures number of pixels change rate (NPCR) and unified average change intensity (UACI) are studied

4.1. Histogram

The histogram of an image is a discrete function that represents the distribution of the number of pixels in an image; according to their intensity of each value, we associate the number of pixels in the image with this level. It indicates for each value between the black (0) and the white (255), how many pixels of this value in the image; in the abscissa (x-axis): the grey level (from 0 to 255); on the ordinate (y-axis): the number of pixels (see **Figure 4**). In a histogram, each vertical bar represents the number of times of level of corresponding grey [11]. For a digitally reliable algorithm, the histogram of the ciphered image must have both properties:

1. The histogram of the ciphered image must be entirely different from the histogram of the original image.

2. To prevent information leakage to an adversary, the histogram of the ciphered image must have a uniform distribution. **Figure 5** shows the histogram of an encrypted image, and we notice that the number of each intentionality (grey level) is close. We find not a higher intensity in a remarkable way or lower remarkably, so the attacker will not be able to have information on the number of the intentionality of the original image.

4.2. The correlation coefficient

The correlation coefficient (CC) determines the relationship and degree of similarity between two variables. In a cryptosystem of images, the correlation is used to measure the difference between two images [4, 12], the relationship between the pixels at the same location in the

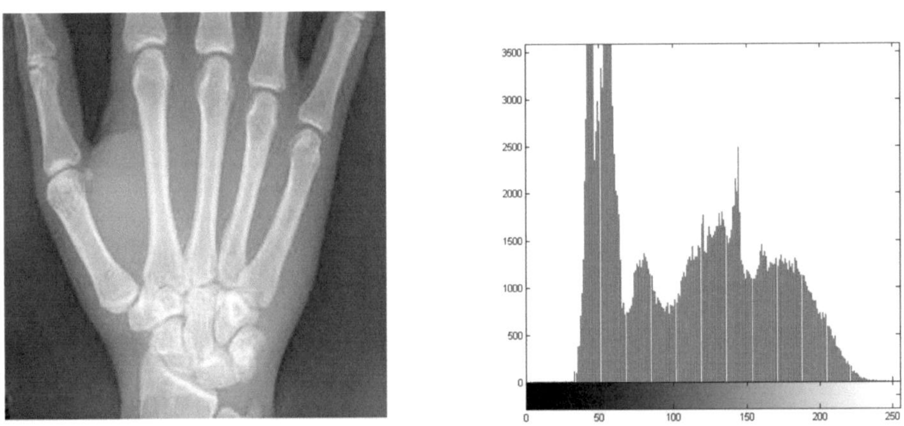

Figure 4. Histogram of greyscale image.

http://dx.doi.org/10.5772/intechopen.75491

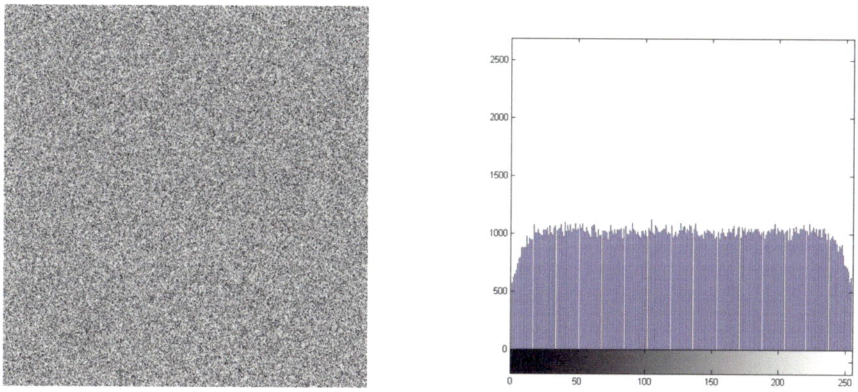

Figure 5. Histogram of ciphered image.

manifest image and the ciphered image. The correlation is a useful measure for judging the quality of the cryptosystem [12, 13].

For a robust cryptosystem, the correlation coefficient (CC) must be very close to zero. Thus, the success of the encryption process signifies small values of CC, and the encrypted image is random and highly uncorrelated [12]. It guarantees that the algorithm is resistant to pixel correlation attack. If the correlation coefficient is close to one, it means that the original image and the ciphered image are very dependent, and the encryption process has failed to hide the details of the original image so that the precise image can be reproduced easily from the encrypted image [12].

The correlation coefficient can be obtained from the formula [11, 12]:

$$CC = \frac{\mathrm{cov}(x,y)}{\sigma_x \sigma_y} = \frac{\sum_{n=1}^{N}(x_i - E(x))(y_i - E(y))}{\sqrt{\sum_{n=1}^{N}(x_i - E(x))^2}\sqrt{\sum_{n=1}^{N}(y_i - E(y))^2}} \tag{1}$$

where x and y are pixel values of the same index of the original image and the ciphered image, respectively.

4.3. Entropy analysis

The entropy of information is another important factor in evaluating the resistance of a cryptographic system. The entropy of the information H (s) of a source s can be calculated by the formula [14]:

$$H(s) = \sum_{n=0}^{2N-1} P(s_i) \log_2 \frac{1}{P(s_i)} \, bits, \tag{2}$$

where the probability of the symbol s_i, in the case of greyscale image is:

$$P(s_i) = \frac{the\ number\ of\ s_i\ in\ the\ ciphered\ image}{2^N} \tag{3}$$

By entropy, we can assess the degree of uncertainty and the randomness of the system [15]. If all the symbols 's_i' have the same probability.

4.4. The irregular deviation

The previous parameters are useful for judging the quality of an algorithm, but they are not good enough because they do not keep any information about pixel positions. A suitable encryption algorithm should change the positions of the pixels randomly and uniformly. This avoids the situation in which some pixels will be subject to a significant change then the other pixels will be subject to a small change [4].

The irregular gap is based on the calculation of the divergence caused by the encryption process [16]. The calculation of the irregular deviation (ID) is summarised in the following steps [4, 12]:

1. Find the matrix D which represents the absolute difference between the value of the pixels before and after the encryption: $D = | I - J |$.
2. Construct the histogram 'H' of the matrix D.
3. Find the average value M_H of the histogram H:

$$M_H = \frac{1}{256}\sum_{i=0}^{256} h_i \tag{4}$$

4. Estimate the absolute difference H_D between the histogram and the average value M_H

$$H_D(i) = | h_i - M_H | \tag{5}$$

5. The irregular deviation (ID) is calculated as follows:

$$ID = \sum_{i=0}^{256} H_D(i) \tag{6}$$

The intermittent deviation (ID) indicates the divergence that has the pixel of the original image [12]. If the irregular deviation is close to a distribution uniform, so this is a good parameter of resistance against statistic attacks [4].

4.5. Noise resistance

Noise is present in most of the images; a good cryptosystem must be robust against noise. If the decrypted image is very similar to the original image, then the encryption system is resistant to noise. To measure the noise, we compare the peak signal-to-noise ratio (PSNR) of the original image and the encrypted image, the PSNR is given by the formula [12]:

$$PSNR = 10 \times \log_{10} \frac{255 \times 255 \times M \times N}{\sum_{i=1}^{M}\sum_{j=1}^{N} (P_{ij} - Q_{ij})^2} (db) \tag{7}$$

where P_{ij} and Q_{ij} are the pixels of line i and column j of the original image and the ciphered image, respectively, M is the number of rows and N is the number of columns of the image.

4.6. NPCR and UACI

In cryptography, diffusion is a desirable property that is introduced by Shannon in his paper published in 1949 [17]. A good cryptosystem must ensure proper dissemination. Diffusion means that if only one bit of the original image is modified, it should entirely unpredictably change the encrypted image. This phenomenon is also called the avalanche effect.

A suitable algorithm must be susceptible to small changes [18]. The hacker can make a little difference in the original image, and then observe the change result. In this way, if the diffusion parameters are low, it can find a significant relationship between the original image and the encrypted image. If the algorithm has an excellent diffusion, the relationship between the encrypted image and the original image is too complicated, and the attacker cannot easily predict the changes. Therefore, this attack would become inefficient.

To measure the difference in a cryptosystem, we modify a bit in the clear image and then calculate the resulting deviation of the encryption process. To test the influence of this change, two measures can be used: NPCR and UACI [11, 12, 19].

We take two encrypted images, C_1 and C_2, the corresponding original images have a single pixel difference. We also define a matrix D that has the same size as C_1 and C_2:

$$D(i,j) = \begin{cases} 0, & if\ C_1(i,j) = C_2(i,j) \\ 1, & if\ C_1(i,j) \neq C_2(i,j) \end{cases} \tag{8}$$

The first measure is the number of pixels change rate (NPCR) is defined by the formula:

$$NPCR = \frac{\sum_{i,j} D(i,j)}{M \times N} \times 100\% \tag{9}$$

where M and N are the width and height of C_1 and C_2, respectively. The NPCR measures the percentage of different pixels in the two images. The NPCR can also be defined by the variance rate of the pixels in the encrypted image caused by the change of a single pixel in the original image.

The second measure is the unified average change intensity (UACI) is defined by:

$$UACI = \frac{1}{M \times N}\left[\sum_{i,j} \frac{C_1(i,j) - C_2(i,j)}{255}\right] \times 100\% \tag{10}$$

5. Cryptology

Significant progress in technology and the enormous amounts of data generated digital births have given rise to new problems. Of these issues, there is data protection or cryptography. Cryptography uses the mathematics to transform a data in the clear into an incomprehensible data, and the opposite direction of this operation is cryptanalysis. Therefore, cryptology has two main branches: cryptography and cryptanalysis. Encryption is the secret writing of information, and cryptanalysis is the analysis of cryptography or the study of the level of security of the systems.

The purpose of cryptography is to provide some security services such as confidentiality, integrity and authenticity [20, 21]. The word cryptography comes from Greek 'Krypto' means I hide and 'graph' means document [22].

Cryptography is not used solely to protect the diplomatic and military communication. Nowadays, image encryption has applications in various fields such as medical and biological image, internet communication, closed-circuit television (CCTV), satellite image, and so on.

In this section, we study the two main branches of cryptology:

5.1. The objectives of cryptography

Cryptography is the study of the techniques used to accomplish the four following purposes [20, 21]: confidentiality, integrity, authentication and nonrepudiation.

Confidentiality: confidentiality is to prohibit access to unauthorised entities.

Integrity: data integrity ensures that information has not been changed between the sender and the receiver.

Authentication: ensure the identity of a person wishing to access this data.

Nonrepudiation (traceability): is to trace any action on the documents. It is a way of preventing an entity from denying participation in an electronic exchange.

5.2. Classification of algorithms

Encryption algorithms can be classified in different ways; according to the structure of the algorithms, depending on the keys or the percentage of the encrypted data [4] (**Figure 6**).

Classification according to the keys: in general, there are three types of encryption systems such as symmetric, asymmetric and hashing:

1. **Symmetric encryption:** also called 'Secret Key Encryption'. The same key is used to write and decrypt, the sender and the recipient must share the same key to perform encryption and decryption. Bob and Alice have to share the secret key via a secure channel to be able to hide the encrypted messages (see **Figure 7**).

2. **Asymmetric encryption:** (public key encryption) is a system where the sender and recipient have a key pair, a public for encryption and a private one for the decryption. Alice uses Bob's public key to encrypt a message for Bob. Bob uses his private key that is not shared to decipher Alice's message (see **Figure 8**).

3. **Hash functions:** a mathematical function that associates a data with a fixed size output is called a hash function. The hash must be unique and short, the return of the hash to the original data must be impossible (see **Figure 9**).

Classification according to the encryption structure: in modern symmetric cryptography, the encryption algorithms can be classified according to the structure into two broad categories: encryption by blocks and stream ciphering.

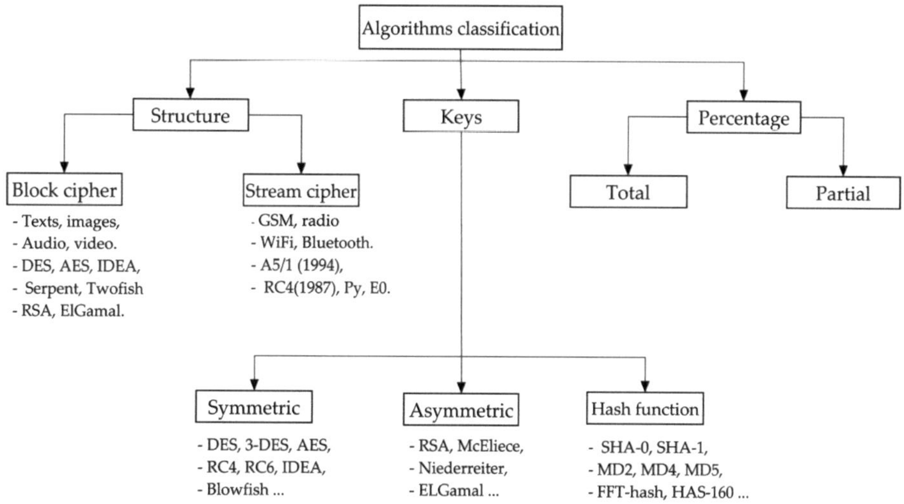

Figure 6. Classification of algorithms.

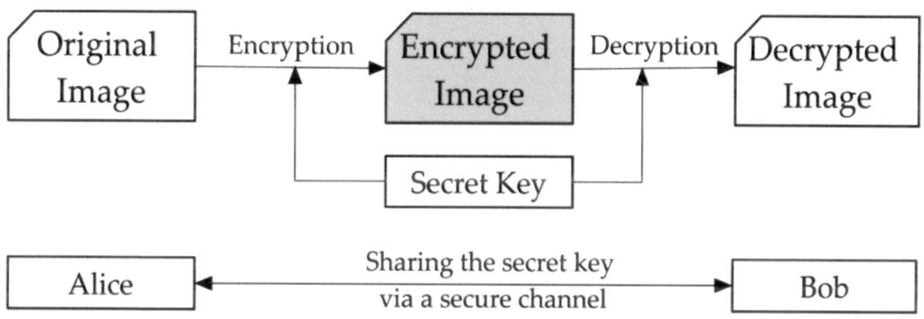

Figure 7. Symmetric encryption.

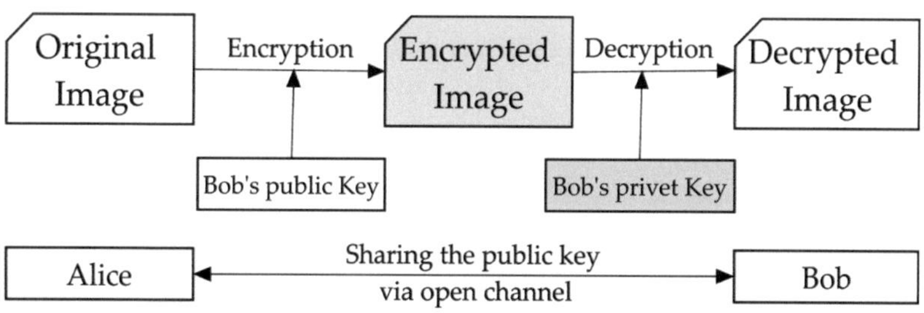

Figure 8. Asymmetric encryption.

1. **Block cypher** has a simple principle, cutting data into blocks fixed size.
2. **Stream cypher**: is to encrypt the bits individually, it is designed to be faster than block cypher and economical regarding resources.

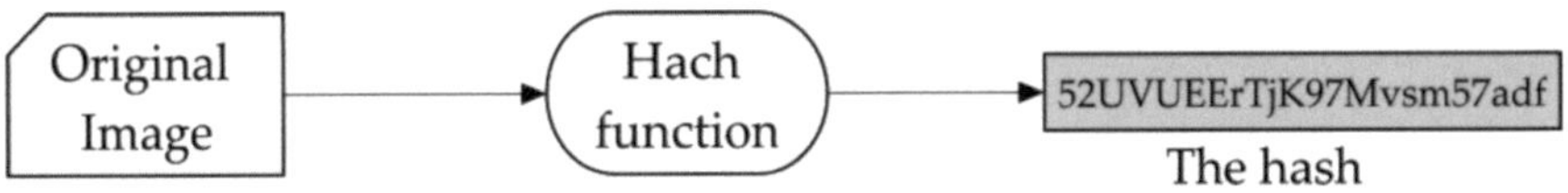

Figure 9. Hash function.

Classification by percentage of encrypted data: depending on the interest of the encrypted data, the encryption can be divided into two groups: total encryption and partial encryption.

1. **Total encryption:** Consists of encrypting all bits of the data, consumes more resources, it is expensive regarding the time of calculation.
2. **Partial encryption:** Or selective is a recent approach that aims to reduce the computing time. It consists of encrypting only a subset of the data. For medical and biological images, to have a reasonable level of confidentiality, at least 12.5% of the data must be encrypted [23, 24].

5.3. Electronic signature

An exciting application of public key cryptography is the digital signature, which is the reverse use of public key encryption. The digital signature is used in the opposite direction of an asymmetric encryption algorithm (**Figure 10**).

5.4. Cryptanalysis

If decryption is to find the precise text knowing the key and the algorithm, cryptanalysis is to try to find the exact version without knowing the key. Cryptanalysis or what Oscar does is the science or art of deciphering encrypted data when the key is unknown. It was developed parallel to cryptography. Among the objectives of cryptanalysis is to measure the weaknesses and robustness of the capacity of a cryptosystem to attack [21, 25].

The primary types of cryptanalysis: According to the information known by the cryptanalysts, we can distinguish the various basic types of cryptanalysis (non-exhaustive list) [21]:

1. **Ciphertext-only attack:** the attacker only has access to encrypted texts of several messages and tries to analyse them to deduce the key or discover the plaintext.

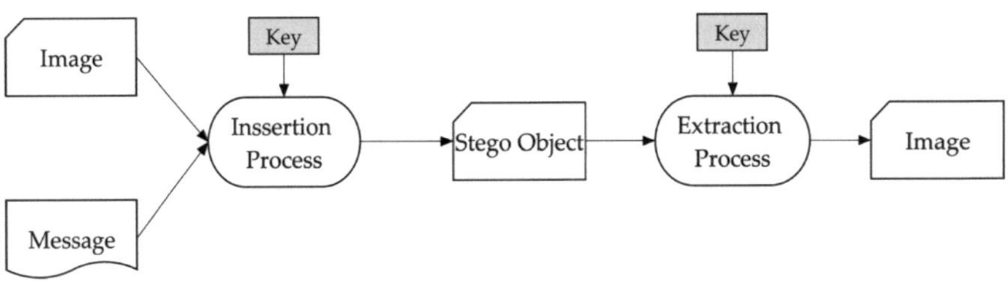

Figure 10. Electronic signature.

2. **Known-plaintext attack:** The adversary knows both parts of the ciphertext and the corresponding plaintext.

3. **Chosen-plaintext attack:** the cryptanalyst has access to the algorithm or the encryption machine, and he/she chooses plain texts and produces the encrypted version of this text. The opponent can use the pairs of clear and encrypted messages to obtain the secret key.

4. **Chosen-ciphertext attack:** The enemy has access to the device of decryption; it has the possibility of choosing the texts to be deciphered without knowing the key.

5. **Brute-force attack:** the attacker tries all combinations of possible keys until the acquisition of the plaintext.

6. Conclusion

In this chapter, we have presented generalities on digital image and medical and biological image, cryptography, primary themes used in encryption, the objectives of cryptography and the classification of algorithms, this ranking is non-exhaustive, there are other types of algorithms like chaotic algorithms [26], as its name suggests, chaotic cryptography relies on the use of chaos. The theory of elliptic curves and the approach of correcting codes are also used to develop new public vital algorithms [27].

We have also mentioned in this chapter the second branch of the cryptology: cryptanalysis, its principles and the different types of attacks. The creation of modern encryption techniques has brought light to new methods of cryptanalysis. We can group these new methods into two large families: differential cryptanalysis [4] and linear cryptanalysis [21].

Graph colouring problem steganography and watermarking can also be a solution to increase safety [12, 24]. Steganography is a technique used to hide secret data in media imperceptibly (**Figure 11**). Many effective steganographic methods can be found in the literature [28]. The primary purpose of watermarking is the protection of copyright by adding visible or nonvisible copyright information. We can find several stenographic techniques [28, 29] and watermarking techniques [30] in the literature.

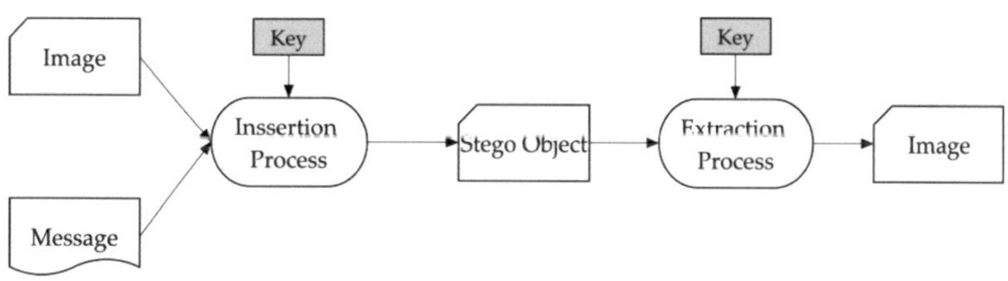

Figure 11. Steganographic scheme

Author details

Abdelkader Moumen

Address all correspondence to: abdelkader.moumen@gmail.com

Department of Mathematics, College of Science, King Khalid University, Abha, Saudi Arabia

References

[1] Gonzalez RC, Woods RE. Digital Image Processing. 2nd ed. Addison-Wesley; 1993

[2] Salles D. Éducation à L'image et aux Médias: La Liberté de la Presse. Centre de Ressources en éducation aux médias CREM; 2005

[3] Gkoulalas-Divanis A, Loukides G. Medical Data Privacy Handbook. Switzerland: Springer International Publishing; 2015. 832 p. ISBN: 978-3-319-23633-9

[4] Moumen A. Imagerie médicale et stockage numériques sécurisées [thesis]. Annaba, Algeria: Badji Mokhtar University; 2017

[5] Calcote S. Developing a secure healthcare information network on the Internet. Healthcare Financial Management. 1997;**51**(1):68

[6] Digital Imaging and Communications in Medicine. http://medical.nema.org/

[7] Integrating the Healthcare Enterprise. http://www.ihe.net/

[8] Health Level Seven. https://www.hl7.org/implement/standards/

[9] Dey S. SD-AEI: An advanced encryption technique for images. In: Second International Conference on Digital Information Processing and Communications (ICDIPC2012). Lithuania: IEEE; 2012. pp. 68-73

[10] Pandey V, Singh A, Shrivastava M. Medical image protection by using cryptography data-hiding and steganography. International Journal of Emerging Technology and Advanced Engineering. 2012;**2**(1):106-109

[11] Li SJ, Chen GR, Zheng X. Chaos-based encryption for digital images and videos. In: Multimedia Security Handbook. 2004

[12] Moumen A, Sissaoui H. Images encryption method using steganographic LSB method, AES and RSA algorithm. Nonlinear Engineering - Modeling and Application. 2016;**6**(1): 53-59. DOI: 10.1515/nleng-2016-0010

[13] Elashry I, Allah O, Abbas A, El-Rabaie S, El-Samie F. Homomorphic image encryption. Journal of Electronic Imaging. 2009;**18**:033002

[14] Han Z, Feng W, Hui L, Da Hai L, Chou L. A new image encryption algorithm based on chaos system. In: 2003 IEEE International Conference on Robotics, Intelligent Systems and Signal Processing. Vol. 2. IEEE; 2003. pp. 778-782

[15] Shu-Jiang X, Ying-Long W, Ji-Zhi W, Min T. A novel image encryption scheme based on chaotic maps. In: 9th International Conference on Signal Processing, 2008 (ICSP 2008); IEEE; 2008. pp. 1014-1018

[16] Ziedan IE, Fouad MM, Salem DH. Application of data encryption standard to bitmap and JPEG images. In: Proceedings of 12th National Radio Science Conference (NRSC2003); 2003. pp. C16/1-C16/8

[17] Shannon C. Communication theory of secrecy systems. Bell System Technical Journal. 1949;**28**(4):656-715

[18] Lian S. Multimedia Content Encryption: Techniques and Applications. London: Taylor & Francis Group, LLC; 2009

[19] Hennelly BM, Sheridan JT. Image encryption based on the fractional Fourier transform. Proceedings of SPIE. 2003;**5202**:76-87

[20] Schneier B. Applied Cryptography. Second ed. New York: John Wiley and Sons; 1996

[21] Stinson D. Cryptography: Theory and Practice. 2nd ed. Boca Raton, USA: Chapman & Hall/CRC; 2002

[22] Singh S. Histoire des Codes Secrets. De l'Égypte des Pharaons à L'ordinateur Quantique. Jean-Claude Lattès; 1999

[23] Spanos GA, Maples TB. Performance study of a selective encryption scheme for the security of networked, real-time video. In: Proceedings of 4th International Conference on Computer Communications and Networks; 1995. pp. 20-23

[24] Moumen A, Bouye M, Sissaoui H. New secure partial encryption method for medical images using graph coloring problem. Nonlinear Dynamics. 2015;**82**(3):1475-1482. DOI: 10.1007/s11071-015-2253-4

[25] Menezes A, van Oorschot P, Vanstone S. Handbook of Applied Cryptography. CRC Press; 1996

[26] Amigó JM. Chaos-based cryptography. In: Intelligent Computing Based on Chaos. Berlin: Springer; 2009. pp. 291-313. ISBN: 978-3-540-95971-7

[27] Miller V. Use of elliptic curves in cryptography in advances in cryptography CRYPTO 85. Lecture Notes in Computer Science. Springer-Verlag. 1989;**218**:417-426. 2, 6

[28] Bender DW, Gruhl NM, Lu A. Techniques for data hiding. IBM Systems Journal. 1996; **35**:313-316

[29] Provos N. Universal Steganography. Août 1998. http://www.outguess.org/

[30] Cayre F, Fontaine C, Furon T. Watermarking security: Theory and practice. IEEE Transactions on Signal Processing. 2005;**53**(10):3976-3987

Chapter 4

Bioinformatics Solutions for Image Data Processing

Pietro Cinaglia, Luciano Caroprese,
Giuseppe Lucio Cascini, Francesco Dattola,
Pasquale Iaquinta, Miriam Iusi, Pierangelo Veltri and
Ester Zumpano

Additional information is available at the end of the chapter

http://dx.doi.org/10.5772/intechopen.76459

Abstract

In recent years, the increasing use of medical devices has led to the generation of large amounts of data, including image data. Bioinformatics solutions provide an effective approach for image data processing in order to retrieve information of interest and to integrate several data sources for knowledge extraction; furthermore, images processing techniques support scientists and physicians in diagnosis and therapies. In addition, bioinformatics image analysis may be extended to support several scenarios, for instance, in cyber-security the biometric recognition systems are applied to unlock devices and restricted areas, as well as to access sensitive data. In medicine, computational platforms generate high amount of data from medical devices such as Computed Tomography (CT), and Magnetic Resonance Imaging (MRI); this chapter will survey on bioinformatics solutions and toolkits for medical imaging in order to suggest an overview of techniques and methods that can be applied for the imaging analysis in medicine.

Keywords: medical imaging, patterns, machine-learning, data-mining

1. Introduction

The image data processing is a relevant support for clinical diagnosis and sharing of health information, for instance, the correct interpretation of images may be crucial for early diseases detection. The use of sophisticated devices has greatly improved the acquisition of data at a very high resolution and faster rate, although the image interpretation process based on machine learning techniques is only recently taking hold. Bioinformatics tools allow to retrieve information able to support a scientist during a diagnosis in order to detect efficiently abnormalities and to monitor their changes over time. In the last years, medical and biological images are quickly growing in terms of size and information content. The term "bioimage" concerns all images related to biological samples acquired using medical technologies such as the Computed Tomography (CT) or the Magnetic Resonance Imaging (MRI); briefly, CT is a technique based on ionizing radiation, for instance, X-rays are used to acquire the images; instead, MRI (or Nuclear-MRI) uses magnetic fields and Radio Frequencies (RF) to produce detailed pictures. An MRI Scanner measures the RF emitted by hydrogen atoms, the RF are directly related to the amount of energy previously provided to the atom and to its necessity to return at an equilibrium state after an excitation. These different approaches make that a CT scanner is better suited to detect cancer or cerebral hemorrhage, while brain tumor is more clearly visible using an MRI scanner. Bioinformatics techniques allow the developing of solutions which provide a support for images acquisition and analysis as well as the integration of biological datasets (e.g., gene data and ontologies) for patterns discovering and disorders detection. For instance, in neuroimaging an interesting branch of study concerns the correlation between brain regions and cognitive functions using several techniques such as the Functional-MRI (fMRI); the latter is based on the Blood Oxygenation Level Dependent (BOLD) signal which represents the increment of blood oxygenation in order to identify the brain region affected during activities (e.g., hands motion) and to reflect the local neuronal signaling [1]. This approach uses the BOLD signal in fMRI to study the activity of the hydrogen atoms that compose the water molecules contained in the brain [2].

BOLD signal in fMRI uses the hydrogen atoms that compose the water molecules contained in the brain to study its activity. An MRI Scanner measures the radio frequency emitted by hydrogen atoms after a first step during which this absorbs energy to the same radio frequency; this effect is related to the necessity of an atom to return to an equilibrium state after an excitation.

When a magnetic field is applied, the atoms absorb energy at a determinate radio frequency; for a clinical-standard fMRI technology at 1.5 Tesla this is approximately 64 MHz. BOLD techniques measure the changes in blood oxygenation resulting from the inhomogeneity of the magnetic field within each small volume of tissue that contains hydrogen atoms. Furthermore, the BOLD signal depends on several magnetic properties, such as Deoxy- and Oxy-hemoglobin. The first introduces an inhomogeneity into the magnetic field due to its paramagnetic properties, the latter is weakly diamagnetic. The variations in the concentrations of Deoxy- and Oxy-hemoglobin produce a decrement and an increment, respectively, in image intensity [3]. Many diseases may be studied using neuroimaging to analyze modifications and alterations in brain regions. Nevertheless, to perform detailed analysis, bioinformatics techniques and algorithms have to be developed. Recent studies focus their attention on the improvement of prediction performance in evaluation of diseases, for instance, in [4] authors recruited 120 schizophrenia patients and 120 healthy controls to compare four methods: Linear Discriminant Analysis (LDA), k-Nearest Neighbors (KNN), Gaussian process classifier (GPC) and Support Vector Machines (SVM). The results illustrate that using brain imaging is possible to study the brain areas as well as a set of specific cognitive functions and their related mental activities. Assuming that a physician needs to develop a model for phenotype–genotype association in Alzheimer's disease (AD), an association study of longitudinal phenotypic markers to AD relevant SNPs could be conducted in order to perform a task-correlated longitudinal sparse regression between MRI and Micro Array technologies, respectively, for the images and the genomic information [5]. The study of bioimaging has met a large quantitative data from heterogeneous sources and the correlation among the data is a decisive step for knowledge extraction; thus, the latter allows a scientist to study novel solutions, and bioinformatics algorithms play a primary role to match heterogeneous sources, based on different models, in order to extract the information of interest.

2. Data formats in biomedical imaging

A file format is a solution able to organize a data inside a file using a specific model to allow the storing and the handling of its information content; building a standard for these processes is necessary to extend the compatibility to the highest number of devices and tools. The increasing adoption in the clinical practice of the 3D solutions, due also to the evolution of technologies in medical imaging such as the Computed Tomography (CT) and the Magnetic Resonance Imaging (MRI), produced the affirmation of the Digital Imaging and Communication in Medicine (DICOM) standard. It is supported from almost all independent manufacturers of imaging equipment that need to guarantee an easy and fast solution for data storage and exchange; furthermore, DICOM is adaptable and extensible to accommodate the requirements for an imaging technology. Briefly, this standard is able to handle the storage, viewing, and transmission of medical images, as well as data sharing in clinical research. In the DICOM format each image is stored in a separate instance (comparable to an 'object' in computer language) which includes metadata and images data. The first contains several information concerning the patient, the manufacturer and technology used to acquire the medical images (modality included), the physician, imaging parameters (e.g., slice thickness and spacing, image orientation and frames features); its size is small as all attributes are represented using raw text in tags-based format. Instead, an image (or slice) concerns the numerical matrices containing a gray-scale value for each related pixel; thus, the volume rendering consisting of the union of all slices in the properly order. In the DICOM standard a redundancy of information is created due to the fact that metadata are repeated in a header generated for all images; this is due to the need to guarantee the independence of each slice from the others both during viewing and transmission. The flexibility of tags information contained in the header produces different information among the scanner manufacturers based on DICOM; this causes incompatibilities and critical failures in the tools that use it.

These disadvantages have led to the implementation of novel standards such as: Neuroimaging Informatics Technology Initiative (NIfTI) standard, Analyze or Minc.

The first version of NIfTI was developed as a set of extensions starting from the Analyze (release 7.5) format in order to extend the support to multidimensional data (e.g., for volumes representation) and to allow the handling of MRI data. Analyze consists of a header (a .hdr file) that contains information (e.g., dimensions and identification), and in voxel raw data (a .img file) for image representation. On the other hand, it does not support the unambiguously establish of the image orientation, as well as the unsigned 16 bits data so its adoption is not widespread [6]. NIfTI is a minimalist format adopted in neuroimaging research consisting, as in Analyze, of a header and an uncompressed image data stored, respectively in a '.hdr' and '.img' file; furthermore, it is able to unify both elements in a single '.nii' file that have the first 348 bytes reserved for the header. In a NIfTI file, an image may be represented using up to seven dimensions of which three are for the space, one for the time and three for the diffusion gradient direction [7]; this feature allowed its growing adoption in neuroscience.

A conversion from DICOM to NIfTI is generally possible using dedicated solutions like 'dcm2nii' (http://www.nitrc.org/projects/dcm2nii/). In [8] a test-scenario based on a cloud implementation of dcm2nii is proposed; it provides the analysis of 812 volumes, stored in 991,000 DICOM files and related to 41 subjects undergoing clinical CT scanners for a neurological study. Experimental results illustrate that the conversion process is extremely time-consuming; in details, authors report that it may need of a computing grid which uses up to 156 cores to process about 52 volumes/minute.

Ultimately, Minc format was developed in 1992 by the Montreal Neurological Institute (MNI); the last release (Minc2) is based on Hierarchical Data Format version 5 (HDF5) and supports large data file as well as a set of tools for DICOM/NIfTI conversion. Each MINC file concerns a multidimensional dataset with all related metadata. It is generally used only in projects developed directly by the MNI Brain Imaging Center for the releasing of library and tools [9].

To date the most widespread formats among the mentioned remain the DICOM and the NIfTI standards which are also supported by most medical device manufacturers.

3. Techniques and methods in medical imaging

Techniques and methods for image analysis are generally based on Machine Learning (ML) and Artificial Intelligence (AI); these allow to efficiently derive relevant information from heterogeneous data such as phenotypes, morphologic features, as well as patterns. In bioinformatics, a pattern may be related to diseases or alterations and it is generally used to associate an image domain with a specific alteration. Briefly, it consists of a sequence of items modeled through a mathematical function able to represent a specific structure, for instance, the patterns can be used to represent a part of an image, or to better say a part of the matrix that contains the value of each pixel/voxel. Assuming that we want to use this approach in neurosciences, a pattern could be used to discover the alterations that affect the normal functions of the brain; the issue could be solved using an algorithm for pattern recognition which is able to integrate information across several sources. In this context, the techniques based on Machine Learning (ML) and Data-Mining approaches are the most used for the developing of bioinformatics tools. Generally, an ML algorithm may be able to identify morphologies by basing its analysis on a training-set of known patterns (supervised learning); alternatively, it could be able to analyze directly an input dataset in order to identify novel pattern using predictions not related to training-sets previously imported but acquired during the analysis (unsupervised learning). Furthermore, a pipeline based on patterns recognition is considered a valid approach for diagnosis and prognosis, as well as to perform studies using several medical imaging from heterogeneous sources. Assuming to conduct a study for the analysis of alterations in a specific brain's region, a pattern recognition solution may be implemented; its pipeline could consist of three main steps: the first able to acquire raw data in a structured model, the second to select the features of interest and the third to perform an algorithm that allow the analysis. The final result will be represented by a set of data with a reduced dimensionality for the space (e.g., represented using the voxel) [10] that will therefore allow to discriminate quickly the patients from the healthy controls using a classifier based, for example, on a cross-validation approach.

In medical image processing, useful approaches are based on the Neural Network (NN). An NN is conceptually inspired by the human brain system and consists of: (i) an input layer, (ii) an output layer and (iii) one or more hidden layers; the number of layers is related to the level of abstraction, as well as to the reliability of the prediction (e.g., a deep neural network hierarchically extends to over 1000 layers). For instance, the NN can be used to extract ROIs [11] using data acquired from mammograms [12]. A powerful set of techniques for learning in NN is the Deep Learning (DL); it is a growing trend for data analysis and medical imaging, becoming one of the breakthrough technologies [13]. A Deep Neural Network performs all possible mappings, importing a dataset built in a previous training step, in order to formulate predictions for the unknown cases in input. Several algorithms based on machine learning are based on DL approaches [14], such as: Convolutional Neural Network (CNN), Deep Neural Network (DNN), Deep Belief Network (DBN), Deep Botlzmann Machine (DBM) and Recurrent Neural Network (RNN); the description and key points are shown in **Table 1**.

Assuming that we want to develop an algorithm to discriminate a specific area (e.g., representing a cancer) from an entire biomedical acquisition, an algorithm for handling of 3D volume and segmentation must be implemented. For instance, UNet [15], VNet and DeepMedic [16], and its improved version DMRes [17], are able to perform a fast and precise segmentation using a CNN architecture for fast and precise segmentation.

In addition, the study of medical sciences (e.g., neurosciences) has met a large quantitative of data and the bioinformatics tools and algorithms play a primary role in reference to knowledge extractions, these allow to perform data-integration techniques obtaining an interdisciplinary view matching heterogeneous sources with different models in order to extract information of interest. In [18] the authors develop BioMediator System to provide a data integration across several biomedical domains and data types in order to allow a biologist to retrieve molecular and genomic information using a browser engine based on head constraints and global path constraints. Assuming that we want to base an application on a mediation approach for a data integration in neurosciences, a first step is related to information retrieving, for instance, the Human Database (HID, http://nbirn.net/research/function/hid.shtm) and the eXtensible Neuroimaging Archive Toolkit (XNAT, http://www.xnat.org) can be used. Subsequently, a query engine for virtual data-integration can be developed. It could implement a OGSA-DAI/DQP architecture, respectively: Open Grid Services Architecture (OGSA) Distributed Access and Integration (DAI) and OGSA Distributed Query Processing (DQP); this solution offers a streaming dataflow workflow evaluation engine, and on a distributed query evaluation engine [19].

Type	Description
Convolutional Neural Network (CNN)	It is based on a neurobiological model that imports 2D inputs in order to produce a 3D output volume for the neuronal activity.
	Generally, it requires large dataset, as well as many layers.
Deep Neural Network (DPN)	DPN is used in non-linear computations using hidden layers (≥2) for classification and regression.
	It is a solution typically used for many areas; its general-purpose approach is very slow not being optimized for a specific context.
Deep Belief Network (DBN)	It uses undirected connections for top two layers in order to allow supervised and unsupervised training for the network.
	For the network initialization perform a layer-by-layer greedy learning; this approach is computationally expensive.
Deep Botlzmann Machine (DBM)	It is based on undirected links among the layers using a stochastic maximum likelihood algorithm.
	Top-Down feedback are supported in order to perform a bust inference.
Recurrent Neural Network (RNN)	It is a Neural Network used for stream data analysis when the output is related to previous computation; during the recursions all weight are shared for all layers. The key points are reported below:
	• Time dependencies modeling
	• Events persistence

Table 1. Deep learning approaches: Key-points and description.

4. Imaging processing solutions

Bioinformatics allows a scientist to extract knowledge from a large set of information consisting of heterogeneous resources, as well as to handle the information of interest and more generally the methods for data storage and retrieval.

For instance, to acquire information of interest from a biomedical image often requires the development of a set of instructions in accordance to the research project; in this regard, a custom algorithm is able to extract knowledge from an input exactly as required by the scientist, and generally more efficiently than a generic commercial or free solution being designed on specific requirements identified in the case study.

Assuming that a researcher wants to implement a solution able to predict structure in accordance with a set of known patterns defined in a "training" phase, a machine-learning approach is perhaps the best choice.

Briefly, the possibilities are mainly two: (i) the implementation of an algorithm "from scratch" or (ii) the importing of existing toolkits (e.g., framework and libraries) within its own algorithm. A development "from scratch" is particularly expensive and time consuming compared to the use of libraries/framework "ready to use". Therefore, it is important to evaluate the availability of existing toolkits before starting the development, as well as the efficiency of those chosen in accordance with the intended aim.

Supposing to use Python as programming-language, Scikit-Learn (http://scikit-learn.org/stable/) is a possible and useful solution for what has been said. It is a general-purpose machine learning library (written in Python) to solve complex data analysis tasks. It uses NumPy and SciPy, respectively, for: (i) storage and manipulation of multi-dimensional array, as well as (ii) for the implementation of data structure and mathematical functions [20]. Scikit-Learn contains also a large set of statistical learning algorithms. Assuming that we want to define a score to identify the variability captured by the model for each voxel then the BOLD signal should be quantified through a regression function. For instance, this approach allows a scientist to analyze fMRI data in order to encode brain activity and decode the related medical images [21].

Alternatively, a useful solution to implement algorithms that use machine-learning techniques for data analysis could be Tensorflow (http://www.tensorflow.org). It is a popular library developed by Google Inc. to implement and execute large-scale artificial neural networks based on typed and multi-dimensional array (named Tensor); a Tensor is a generalization of arrays and matrices with higher size. Its approach is based on nodes defined during a training task, in each training iteration new links are established.

Furthermore, Tensorflow's API allows the implementation of tools able to train and to test neural networks using computational graphs built in Python or C++. Assuming that a scientist wants to develop a machine-learning interface than the TensorFlow's API is a good starting point, for instance, the DICOM support may be extended in order to implement a classifier for medical imaging that uses bioimage datasets as input for tensors [22]. Therefore, this solution could therefore represent a potential tool useful for diagnostic in the clinical practice. Assuming that we want to improve the accuracy of a disease diagnosis, a deep learning solution may be implemented. For instance, the input for the model could be represented by Alzheimer's Disease Neuroimaging Initiative (ADNI) data acquired with Magnetic Resonance Imaging (MRI) or Positron Emission Tomography (PET) techniques. To evaluate the model a pre-processing step is performed in order to (i) correct the intensity inhomogeneity, (ii) normalize data into a template space, (iii) define maps for the gray matter tissue and (iv) improve the signal-to-noise ratio (e.g., using a Gaussian kernel). An interesting requirement could be represented by the possibility of capturing the highly nonlinear relationships between Input and Output; the Convolutional Neural Networks (CNNs) are a candidate solution for this aim (as previously defined: *a CNN is based on a neurobiological model that imports 2D inputs in order to produce a 3D output volume for the neuronal activity. Generally, it requires large dataset, as well as many layers*). In [23], a similar approach is developed: the authors focused on evaluating of a CNN model for image data completion. The solution is based mainly on two steps: (i) complete the missing data using CNN (a comparison with other methods based on KNN and Zero is evaluated); (ii) estimate the performance using a l2-norm regularized logistic regression classifiers on the output. In the experiments, the data are randomly divided into two sub-sets, respectively, one-third for the tests and two-thirds for the training step; in the latter, a CNN model is built in order to retrieve the nonlinear relationship between different data modalities in the network. In accordance with the authors the results show that the predicted data (obtained from PET images) can potentially be used to improve the accuracy of disease diagnosis.

4.1. Toolkits in medical imaging

More toolkits are available from several program languages and platforms in bioinformatics, and generally, these are based on Machine Learning (ML) solutions (or similar approaches). A standard which is able to produce a comparison among toolkits in ML is not defined, as each tool is often designed for determinate needs related to different problems, and its approach is therefore to be considered context-specific [24].

A list of useful toolkits is shown below and summarized in **Table 2**; only objective criteria (e.g., programming-language and features) are reported so that everyone may correlate a toolkit in reference to their needs.

- ODTbrain is a Python library that implements a back-propagation algorithm for dense diffraction tomography in 3D [25]. The three-dimensional (3D) refractive index distribution of a unique cell allows to describe its inner structure in a marker-free manner. The term dense, full-view tomographic data set denotes a set of images of a cell acquired for multiple rotational positions, densely distributed from 0 to 360 degrees. The projection tomography, based on the inversion of the Radon transform, is generally used to perform the reconstruction and its quality is greatly improved when first order scattering is taken into account. This advanced reconstruction technique is called diffraction tomography. The first implementation of diffraction tomography has been proposed in ODTbrain. The algorithm is an extension to optical projection tomography that takes into account diffraction of light due to the refractive index of the sample. In ODTbrain the reconstruction process is divided into three main steps: filtering, reconstruction and object data construction. ODTbrain is able to reconstruct 3D refractive index maps from projections of biological or artificial phase objects; the algorithm is validated performing the analysis on a simulated dataset and subsequently authors have compared results with the reconstruction qualities of Optical Diffraction Tomography (ODT) and Optical Projection Tomography (OPT).

Name	Language	Main methods
jicbioimage	Python	Microscopy data, view and explore data, generate reproducible analyses.
Scikit-Learn	Python	Classification, regression, clustering, model selection, preprocessing.
ODTbrain	Python	Back-propagation algorithm for dense diffraction tomography in 3D.
CP-CHARM	Python	Image automated classification (optimization is not required).
SCIFIO	Java	Handling of scientific images.
NIF	(framework, web-based)	Queries support for NIF.
WHIDE	(web-based)	H2SOM clustering, imaging analysis (space and collocation).
GALA	Python	Data acquisition and analysis in neurophysiology.
ACQ4	Python	Experiments automation.

Table 2. Toolkits for medical imaging.

- CP-CHARM [26] is a user-friendly image-based classification algorithm. It is inspired by WND-CHARM. The latter is a multi-purpose image classification algorithm that can be applied without optimization or modifying the starting data; features are computed on the whole image and no segmentation is required [27]. Using the CP-CHARM algorithm a user is able to extract several morphological features from an image without first being segmented; furthermore, in order to be suitable and accessible to all the biological research community, even with few expertise, CP-CHARM relies on CellProfiler an open source image analysis software for quantitative analysis of biological images [28]. The proposed method has been demonstrated to perform well on a wide range of bioimage classification problems. The proposed method has been validated firstly by showing that it could achieve performance similar to those of WND-CHARM. Then the algorithm has been used on several kinds of biological datasets, for example, data freely available from the Broad Bioimage Benchmark Collection (BBBC) [29] and tissue images from the Human Protein Atlas (HPA) [30]. CP-CHARM has been demonstrated to perform well on a wide range of bioimage classification problems.

- SCIFIO is a flexible framework for SCientific Image Format Input and Output. In other words, it is a library for reading and writing N-dimensional image data. SCIFIO is an open source plugin for the SciJava framework that offers support for handling of scientific images. SCIFIO defines a common pattern for image format construction and can be easily extended—from custom formats to new metadata schema. It is developed by the ImageJ development team at the Laboratory for Optical and Computational Instrumentation (LOCI) at the University of Wisconsin-Madison. The Open Microscopy Environment's Bio-Formats library provides the ability to convert many proprietary image formats to a common OME-TIFF format, using the OME-XML schema. This allows scientists to freely share image data without being restricted by proprietary format barriers. It is part of the SciJavasoftware stack and in use by several projects including ImageJ2, ImgLib2, and the Insight Toolkit (ITK). One of the main features of SCIFIO concerns the support of multiple domain-specific formats within a unified environment [31].

- The Neuroscience Information Framework (NIF) is a framework that promotes the integrating access to Web-Based neuroscience resources [32]. It is supported from the Institutes and Centers forming the NIH Blueprint for Neuroscience Research. The framework is based on an Open Source design and offers dynamic and web-accessible resources focused on neuroscience that are described using an integrated terminology, also it is able to support concept-based queries as well as the integration of neuroscience information with complementary areas of biomedicine.

- Web-based Hyperbolic Image Data Explorer (WHIDE) combines more features related to principles of machine learning and scientific-information in order to analyze the aspects (space and collocation) of Toponome Imaging System (TIS) images. WHIDE uses Hierarchical Hyperbolic SOM (H2SOM) clustering to resolve non-linear features and dynamic interactive manipulation of the colors, as well as to organize the clusters in a hierarchical structure. Authors tested the tool for TIS analysis but is not excluded that it is applicable to other MBI data [33].

- Graph-based Active Learning of Agglomeration (GALA) is an algorithm, implemented in python language, for image segmentation. GALA belongs to a class of segmentation algorithms called agglomerative algorithms, in which segments are formed by merging smaller segments. It works by repeatedly consulting a gold standard segmentation (prepared by human annotators) as it agglomerates sub-segments according to its current best guess. More specifically, GALA accumulates a training dataset used to fit a classifier that guides the subsequent agglomeration decisions. GALA includes several scientific Python libraries: numpy, scipy and others, to perform segmentation analysis; also, it implements a solution based on machine-learning approach [34].
- ACQ4 is a modular software for data acquisition and analysis in neurophysiology research. It is available for download at http://www.acq4.org. ACQ4 integrates the task of acquiring, managing and analyzing experimental data. It is developed as general-purpose tools with the main aim to combine traditional electrophysiology, photostimulation and imaging for experiments automation. The system is highly modular and therefore it is quite simple to add new functionalities.

In [35] authors present several use-cases for ACQ4 to illustrate its functionalities reported as a set of experiments that are possible using this tool; below are briefly listed: (i) Multiphoton calcium imaging during whisker deflection; (ii) Laser scanning photostimulation; (iii) In vitro patch clamp with drug perfusion and (iv) In vivo recording during an operant conditioning task. ACQ4 uses free and open-source tools such as Python, NumPy/SciPy for numerical computation, PyQt for the user interface and PyQtGraph for scientific graphics. ACQ4.

- jicbioimage is a tool implemented in python language for automated and reproducible bioimage analysis; jicbioimage has been used on over 15 internal projects at various stages of the publication pipeline [36]. Using jicbioimaget an user is able to (i) read bioimage data in several format, for this aim the features of Python-BioFormat are imported by authors; (ii) transform and segment images using methods based on numpy, scipy, and scikit-image and (iii) examine the versions for an experiment: briefly, the versions for an initial image are stored by jicbioimage during all transformations to help a scientist to understands the steps performed by the tool and its sub-processes.
- eIMES 3D (standing for Evolution Imaging System 3D for Mobile) is a system that supports image reconstruction with dedicated features for the mobile environments [37, 38]. Using eIMES 3D, a cancer network data infrastructure can be defined and implemented in order to integrate information regarding rare and complex diseases. Furthermore, it provides a hardware infrastructure to connect multiple devices, as well as to create workstations (WorkSpaces) with independent and asynchronous features for information retrieving in order to acquire 3D images from a central database. Briefly, eIMES 3D allows:
    - full control and management of data and imaging by means of artificial intelligence algorithms;
    - advanced stereoscopic 3D visualization by using theWebGL innovative technology;

http://dx.doi.org/10.5772/intechopen.76459

- sharing of medical data;
- distribution of 3D imaging on different output devices;
- query the system through a search of the various case studies.

The AI algorithms allow to provide a new layer of information by applying set of rules fixed by international protocols, or by expert of the domain. These conceptually use known information and a set of production rules to derive new information or to change beliefs as a result of new knowledge. The logical formalization of AI algorithm is defined using a set of logical rules in order to extract new layers deriving knowledge (deductive process). Furthermore, the AI algorithms can apply an abductive process: using novel observation, that modifies the existing protocol, the information can be updated with the new specifications.

5. Conclusion

The fast growth of medical imaging may be seen monitoring the increase of available solutions and the interest in its research field, as well as in clinical practice. The increasing adoption in the clinical practice of the 3D solutions, due also to the evolution of technologies in medical imaging, such as the Computed Tomography and the Magnetic Resonance Imaging, produced a large amount of data. Knowledge extraction from medical images is still a complex task; this chapter recalls several images techniques and approaches used in bioinformatics, also describing some useful toolkits for the development of custom solutions.

Author details

Pietro Cinaglia[1], Luciano Caroprese[2], Giuseppe Lucio Cascini[1], Francesco Dattola[3], Pasquale Iaquinta[3], Miriam Iusi[3], Pierangelo Veltri[1] and Ester Zumpano[2]*

*Address all correspondence to: e.zumpano@deis.unical.it

1 Department of Surgical and Medical Sciences, Magna Graecia University of Catanzaro, Italy

2 Department of Informatics, Modeling, Electronics and System Engineering, University of Calabria, Italy

3 e way Enterprise Business Solutions Cosenza, Italy

References

[1] Matthews P, Jezzard P. Functional magnetic resonance imaging. Journal of Neurology, Neurosurgery, and Psychiatry. 2004;**75**(1):6-12

[2] Tang Y, Meng L, Wan CM, et al. Identifying the presence of Parkinson's disease using lowfrequency fluctuations in BOLD signals. Neuroscience Letters. 2017;**645**:1-6

[3] Heeger DJ, Ress D. What does fMRI tell us about neuronal activity? Nature Reviews Neuroscience. 2002;**3**(2):142-151

[4] Li Z, Wang Y, Quan W, Wu T, Lv B. Evaluation of different classification methods for the diagnosis of schizophrenia based on functional near-infrared spectroscopy. Journal of Neuroscience Methods. 2015;**241**:101-110

[5] Wang H, Nie F, Huang H, et al. From phenotype to genotype: An association study of longitudinal phenotypic markers to Alzheimer's disease relevant SNPs. Bioinformatics. 2012;**28**(18):i619-i625

[6] Larobina M, Murino L. Medical image file formats. Journal of Digital Imaging. 2014;**27**(2): 200-206

[7] Li X, Morgan PS, Ashburner J, Smith J, Rorden C. The first step for neuroimaging data analysis: DICOM to NIfTI conversion. Journal of Neuroscience Methods. 2016;**264**:47-56

[8] Bao S, Plassard AJ, Landman BA, Gokhale A. Cloud engineering principles and technology enablers for medical image processing-as-a-Service. Proceeding of IEEE International Conference on Cloud Engineering. 2017;**2017**:127-137

[9] Vincent RD, Neelin P, Khalili-mahani N, et al. MINC 2.0: A flexible format for multimodal Images. Frontiers in Neuroinformatics. 2016;**10**:35

[10] Haller S, Lovblad KO, Giannakopoulos P, Van de ville D. Multivariate pattern recognition for diagnosis and prognosis in clinical neuroimaging: State of the art, current challenges and future trends. Brain Topography. 2014;**27**(3):329-337

[11] Sonka M, Hlavac V, Boyle R. Image Processing, Analysis and Machine Vision. 1995. 10.1007/978-1-4899-3216-7

[12] Sahiner B, Chan HP, Petrick N, et al. Classification of mass and normal breast tissue: A convolution neural network classifier with spatial domain and texture images. IEEE Transactions on Medical Imaging. 1996;**15**(5):598-610

[13] MIT Technology Review. 2013 [Online]. Available https://www.technologyreview.com/s/513696/deep-learning

[14] Ravi D, Wong C, Deligianni F, et al. Deep Learning for Health Informatics. IEEE Journal of Biomedical and Health Informatics. 2017;**21**(1):4-21

[15] Ourselin S, Joskowicz L, Sabuncu MR, et al. Medical Image Computing and Computer-Assisted Intervention – MICCAI. 2016, 19th International Conference, Athens, Greece, October 17-21, 2016, Proceedings. Springer; 2016

[16] Kamnitsas K, Ledig C, Newcombe VFJ, Simpson JP, Kane AD, Menon DK, Rueckert D, Glocker B. Efficient multi-scale 3D CNN with fully connected CRF for accurate brain lesion segmentation. Medical Image Analysis. 2017;**36**(1):61-78

[17] Kamnitsas K, Ferrante E, Parisot S, Ledig C, Nori AV, Criminisi A, Rueckert D, Glocker B. DeepMedic for brain tumor segmentation. In: Crimi A, Menze B, Maier O, Reyes M, Winzeck S, Handels H, editors. BrainLes 2016. LNCS, vol. 10154, pp. 138-149

[18] Wang K, Tarczy-Hornoch P, Shaker R, Mork P, Brinkley JF. BioMediator data integration: beyond genomics to neuroscience data. In: American Medical Informatics Association Annual Symposium Proceedings; 2005. pp. 779-783

[19] Wang L, Alpert KI, Calhoun VD, Cobia DJ, Keator DB, King MD, Kogan A, Landis D, Tallis M, Turner MD, Potkin SG, Turner JA, Ambite JL. SchizConnect: Mediating neuroimaging databases on schizophrenia and related disorders for large-scale integration. Neuroimage. Jan 2016;**124**:1155-1167

[20] Pedregosa F, Varoquaux G, Gramfort A, Michel V, Thirion B, Grisel O, Blondel M, Prettenhofer P, Weiss R, Dubourg V, Vanderplas J, Passos A, Cournapeau D, Brucher M, Perrot M, Duchesnay E. Scikit-learn: Machine learning in Python. Journal of Machine Learning Research. 2011;**12**:2825-2830

[21] Abraham A, Pedregosa F, Eickenberg M, et al. Machine learning for neuroimaging with scikit-learn. Frontiers in Neuroinformatics. 2014;**8**:14

[22] Zhang YC, Kagen AC. Machine Learning Interface for Medical Image Analysis. Journal of Digital Imaging. 2017;**30**(5):615-621

[23] Li R, Zhang W, Suk HI, Wang L, Li J, Shen D, Ji S. Deep learning based imaging data completion for improved brain disease diagnosis. Medical Image Computing and Computer-Assisted Intervention. 2014;**17**(Pt 3):305-312

[24] Erickson BJ, Korfiatis P, Akkus Z, Kline T, Philbrick K. Toolkits and Libraries for Deep Learning. Journal of Digital Imaging. 2017;**30**(4):400-405

[25] Muller P, Schurmann M and Guck J. ODTbrain: a Python library for full-view, dense diffraction tomography. BMC Bioinformatics. 2015;**16**:367:1-367:9

[26] Uhlmann V, Singh S, Carpenter AE. CP-CHARM: segmentation-free image classification made accessible. BMC Bioinformatics. 2016;**17**:51

[27] Orlov N, Shamir L, Macura T, Johnston J, Eckley DM, Goldberg IG. WND-CHARM: Multi-purpose image classification using compound image transforms. Pattern Recognition Letters. 2008;**29**(11):1684-1693

[28] Dao D, Fraser AN, Hung J, Ljosa V, Singh S, Carpenter AE. Cell Profiler Analyst: interactive data exploration, analysis and classification of large biological image sets. Bioinformatics. 2016

[29] Ljosa V, Sokolnicki KL, Carpenter AE. Annotated high-throughput microscopy image sets for validation. Nature Methods. 2012;**9**(7):637

[30] Uhlen M, Oksvold P, Fagerberg L, Lundberg E, Jonasson K, Forsberg M, et al. Towards a knowledge-based human protein atlas. Nature Biotechnology. 2010;**28**(12):1248-1250

[31] Hiner MC, Rueden CT, Eliceiri KW. SCIFIO: An extensible framework to support scientific image formats. BMC Bioinformatics. 2016;**17**(1):521

[32] Gardner D, Akil H, Ascoli GA, et al. The neuroscience information framework: a data and knowledge environment for neuroscience. Neuroinformatics. 2008;**6**(3):149-160

[33] Kölling J, Langenkämper D, Abouna S, Khan M, Nattkemper TW. WHIDE–a web tool for visual data mining colocation patterns in multivariate bioimages. Bioinformatics. 2012;**28**(8):1143-1150

[34] Nunez-iglesias J, Kennedy R, Plaza SM, Chakraborty A, Katz WT. Graph-based active learning of agglomeration (GALA): A Python library to segment 2D and 3D neuroimages. Frontiers in Neuroinformatics. 2014;**8**:34

[35] Campagnola L, Kratz MB, Manis PB. ACQ4: An open-source software platform for data acquisition and analysis in neurophysiology research. Frontiers in Neuroinformatics. 2014;**8**:3

[36] Olsson TS, Hartley M. jicbioimage: A tool for automated and reproducible bioimage analysis. PeerJ. 2016;**4**:e2674

[37] Iaquinta P, Iusi M, Caroprese L, Turano S, Palazzo S, Dattola F, Pellegrino I, Veltri P, Zumpano E. eIMES 3D: An innovative medical images analysis tool to support diagnostic and surgical intervention. Procedia Computer Science. 2017;**110**:459-464

[38] Turano S, Biamonte R, Zumpano E, Veltri P, Confessore G, Dattola F, Pellegrino I, Iaquinta P, Iusi M, De Stefano R, Romeo F, Palazzo S. ReCaTuR, Rare Cancer Network Calabria, Implementing a software system based on showing of 3D stereoscopic imaging data. Annals of Oncology. 2016;**27**(suppl 4):iv100-iv100

Chapter 5

Abnormal Tissue Zone Detection and Average Active Stress Estimation in Patients with LV Dysfunction

Sareh Behdadfar, Laurent Navarro, Joakim Sundnes, Molly Maleckar, Hans Henrik Odland and Stephane Avril

Additional information is available at the end of the chapter

http://dx.doi.org/10.5772/intechopen.75202

Abstract

Detection of regional ventricular dysfunction is a challenging problem. This study presents an efficient method based on ultrasound (US) imaging and finite element (FE) analysis, for detecting akinetic and dyskinetic regions in the left ventricle (LV). The underlying hypothesis is that the contraction of a healthy LV is approximately homogeneous. Therefore, any deviations between the image-based measured deformation and a homogeneous contraction FE model should correspond to a pathological region. The method was first successfully applied to synthetic data simulating an acute ischemia; it demonstrated that the pathological areas were revealed with a higher contrast than those observed directly in the deformation maps. The technique was then applied to a cohort of eight left bundle branch block (LBBB) patients. For this group, the heterogeneities were significantly less pronounced than those revealed for the synthetic cases but the method was still able to identify the abnormal regions of the LV. This study indicated the potential clinical utility of the method by its simplicity in a patient-specific context and its ability to quickly identify various heterogeneities in LV function. Further studies are required to determine the model accuracy in other pathologies and to investigate its robustness to noise and image artifacts.

Keywords: acute ischemia, left ventricle, cardiac mechanics, GE Healthcare US, EchoPac®

1. Introduction

Realistic finite element (FE) simulation of regional defects caused by pathologies such as acute ischemia remains a significant problem for physiologically based FE analysis of the heart.

From the moment that the cell death starts to the thinning and the expansion of the scar surface of myocardium tissue, it takes approximately 21 days before the remodeling phase starts [1]. Therefore, an accessible method to detect and characterize the influenced region can provide a better plan for diagnosis of these patients with medications and myocardial injection to avoid tissue progressive remodeling [2, 3].

Tracking the deformation of the LV has been actively pursued for the last decades, but important information is lacking about in-vivo wall stress reconstruction in medical imaging modalities for computational purpose [4]. Accurate FE models based on high-resolution medical images can be applied for stress reconstruction, but these models are still limited to medical research and not generally available in the clinic.

Generally, the primary tool for ischemia detection is the analysis of standard electrocardiogram (ECG) signals. The majority of research focus regarding mathematical and computational tools of ischemic zone detection were addressed by electro-physiology models [5–8]. An alternative method for ischemia detection is to assess cardiac function with magnetic resonance imaging (MRI) modalities. However, the abnormal zone detection in MRI modalities is limited and remains a challenging problem [9–11]. In this context, the speckle tracking technique which employs the non-invasive ultrasound (US) [12] has become a commonplace technique in clinical daily practice [13] due to the accessibility of this system.

In this chapter, we study the possibilities of computing a region of abnormal function from 4D strain acquired with the EchoPac® system. The strain estimates are based on speckle tracking, and capture 3D strain through time for 17 LV regions based on the standardized segments of the American Heart Association (AHA) [14].

Coupling US data with computations based on the FE method may provide more detailed information about the mechanical state of the patient's heart. The purpose of the present chapter is to apply FE simulations to detect regions of abnormal function in the LV, based on the hypothesis that a homogeneous contraction is a regional assumption for a healthy LV, and large deviations between measured deformations and FE simulations based on homogeneous contraction will correspond to an abnormal region. We aim to investigate the validity of this hypothesis using the 4D strain data acquired with EchoPac®.

The chapter is organized as follows. First, we present an overview of our pipeline and of the equations for the systolic phase of the heart cycle. Next, we test the accuracy of the method using synthetic data, simulating zones of acute ischemia in the LV. Finally, the methodology is applied to a cohort of patients with left bundle branch block (LBBB), and we discuss the results and the strengths and limitations of the proposed method.

2. Material and method

Akinetic or dyskinetic regions such as ischemic regions or infarcts may be detected in medical images as regions of abnormal deformation. However, healthy tissue surrounding a pathological region may also show abnormal patterns of deformation, which makes it challenging to locate the pathological region. The purpose of the present paper is to investigate an alternative method for detecting abnormal regions, by comparing measured strains with strains resulting from a homogeneous contraction. As noted earlier, the underlying hypothesis is that the healthy contraction is approximately homogeneous [15, 16], and the largest deviation will therefore be associated with the pathological region. To test our hypothesis, we propose to:

1. Build a patient-specific mesh from the images (using an in-house mesh morphing method [17]),
2. Apply a uniform contraction and tune this to give the closest match to the patient's strain data,
3. Evaluate the spatial deviations, and compare the region of largest deviation to the (known) regions of abnormalities.

These main steps of the methodology are illustrated in **Figure 1**. When applying the algorithm to the patient data, it is necessary to generate a patient-specific FE mesh for each individual case. Besides, the accuracy of the geometry associated with the generic LV model is greater than the patient-specific geometries, hence, the need to adapt the generic model to each patient. This task is accomplished by a previously developed mesh morphing method, which takes a generic LV mesh and adapts it to the patients' image data [17]. The rest of the methodology consists of a minimization loop on the active tension a_f. For each patient-specific mesh, the algorithm assumes a constant value for the actively generated stress, denoted as average active stress (AAS), and performs a systolic FE simulation. Then, the resulting regional strains are compared with the patient's data, and a minimization procedure is performed to minimize the deviation between measured and simulated regional strains. The final, minimized, deviation is then visualized and analyzed in order to locate regions of dysfunctional LV segments.

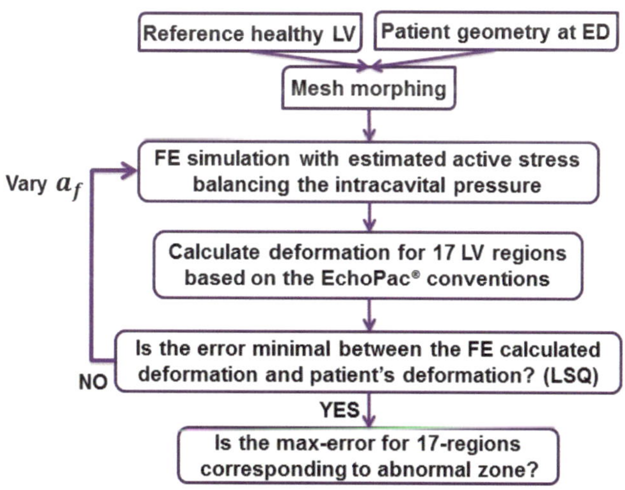

Figure 1. The developed patient-specific pipeline. First, we morph a reference FE mesh to the patient data, and then we estimate an average active stress (AAS) to minimize the deviations between FE simulation and the patient data using sum of squared differences (LSQ). a_f is the active tension. Finally, we compare these results to detect the abnormal zone.

The main reason why we focus on the systolic phase is that in acute ischemia, the passive behavior of the abnormal zone during diastolic phase stays intact, whereas the first appearance of the defected region is during the active contraction [4]. As a result, remodeling of abnormal tissue induces a different deformation due to the average stress in regional LV motion.

2.1. Reference FE simulation model for systolic phase

To examine the abnormal tissue size effects on global and regional deformation, we need to explain the model which was used for FE systolic phase. We employed a healthy volunteer LV extracted from 4D US [18] at end diastole (ED). A 3D mesh with eight-noded linear hexahedral elements was created using Abaqus® mesh generation software. The reference mesh had 155,172 nodes and 141,405 elements.

To incorporate the known material anisotropy of the LV during the systolic phase, we defined a local curvilinear coordinate system aligned with the local fibre orientation, to model myocyte contraction [19, 20]. We assumed a helical fibre distribution, with a helical angle varying from -70° at the epicardial surface to 60° at the endocardial surface (0° is the circumferential direction). At each point, we defined the local orthonormal basis as $(\vec{\mathbf{e}}_n, \vec{\mathbf{e}}_s, \vec{\mathbf{e}}_f)$, where $(\vec{\mathbf{e}}_f)$ is aligned with the local fibre [21].

We were interested in computing the mechanical state of the tissue at ES. The tissue deformation in the systolic phase results from a combination of active and passive mechanical properties. We modeled this interaction using a so-called active stress approach, where the total tissue stress is decomposed into an active ($\sigma_{\mathbf{active}}$) and a passive ($\sigma_{\mathbf{passive}}$) part.

$$\sigma_{total} = \sigma_{passive} + \sigma_{active}. \tag{1}$$

Introducing $\mathbf{R}_f$ as the matrix of transformation from global to local coordinate system, $\mathbf{F}$ as the deformation gradient, and $J = det(\mathbf{F})$ ($J = 1$ for incompressible tissue), the active stress in global coordinates can be expressed as

$$\sigma_{\mathbf{active}} = J^{-1}\mathbf{F}\mathbf{R}_f^{-1}\begin{bmatrix} 0 & 0 & 0 \\ 0 & 0 & 0 \\ 0 & 0 & a_f \end{bmatrix}\mathbf{R}_f\mathbf{F}^T, \tag{2}$$

where a_f is the active tension developed by the contracting fibres.

Following our assumption of homogeneous contraction, the value of a_f is assumed constant in space, and is tuned to provide the best possible match with the measured strain data for each patient. The chosen maximum value for a_f was set to 135 kPa [22, 23]. The passive component in Eq. (1) was modeled as hyperelastic, with stress derived from a strain energy function W;

$$\sigma_{\mathbf{passive}} = J^{-1}\mathbf{F}(\partial W/\partial \mathbf{E})\mathbf{F}^T. \tag{3}$$

Here $\mathbf{E}$ is the Green–Lagrange deformation tensor.

http://dx.doi.org/10.5772/intechopen.75202

In the literature, different strain energy functions have been proposed for the cardiac tissue [24–26]. To reduce the complexity and number of parameters in the model, and based on the assumption that at ES the tissue stress is dominated by the active component, we used a simple Mooney-Rivlin strain energy model, as previously used by Marchesseau et al. [27]:

$$W = c_1\left(\bar{I}_1 - 3\right) + c_2\left(\bar{I}_2 - 3\right) + K(J - 1)^2. \tag{4}$$

Here c_1, c_2 are material parameters (MPs), $\bar{I}_1$ and $\bar{I}_2$ are the invariants of the right Cauchy-Green tensor and $K = 2/d_1$ is the bulk modulus.

We performed a reference FE simulation using the following MPs: c_1 = 0.0187 MPa, c_2 = 0.0198 MPa, d_1 = 0.1697 MPa, and the contraction model outlined earlier. The boundary conditions were as follows: a pressure of 11.24 kPa was applied to the endocardial surface [23], the epicardial surface was unloaded, and the basal nodes were assigned to remain coplanar during deformation [27]. This reference FE simulation was compared with results reported by Dorri et al. [23] and showed good agreement in terms of LV ejection fraction (EF) (33.83%), wall thickness change (18.7%) and Von Mises stresses, which are in the range of 100–150 kPa [23, 28–30].

We used these boundary conditions, MPs and contraction model for the *patient-specific* FE simulations of the provided cohort with the Abaqus® software solver.

2.2. Application on synthetic acute ischemia

Two reference meshes have been used for application of our developed pipeline.

2.2.1. Ellipsoid reference mesh

A truncated ellipsoid mesh has been generated using Abaqus® software. The height of the mesh was 9 cm, and the wall thickness was 1 cm. The fibre directions were assigned as outlined earlier. We defined a small zone at the equatorial level of the septal wall (see **Figure 2**) as acutely ischemic, i.e. non-contractile. The active stress in this region was set to zero, while the rest of the reference FE model, a_f = 160 kPa, was attributed. The same condition as explained in Section 2.1 in terms of boundary conditions, ES pressure, contraction model and MPs was used to perform this model. In order to relate the results to the echo images, we defined a midwall surface mesh that was split into 17 segments as shown in **Figure 3** [14]. We will refer to this mesh as the midwall mesh throughout this chapter. Regional deformations were calculated as average strains in each segments (longitudinal, circumferential and area strain), similar to the output of the EchoPac strain analysis.

To provide a first test of the hypothesis underlying this research, we performed an FE simulation with an AAS, and tuned the active stress parameter to match the strains of the synthetic reference model as closely as possible. The cost function was defined as the sum of the squared differences (LSQ) between the AAS strains and the reference strains, and a simple minimization was performed by gradually increasing a_f from 90 to 180 kPa in 5 kPa steps. The smallest cost function obtained with this procedure was used as the closest match.

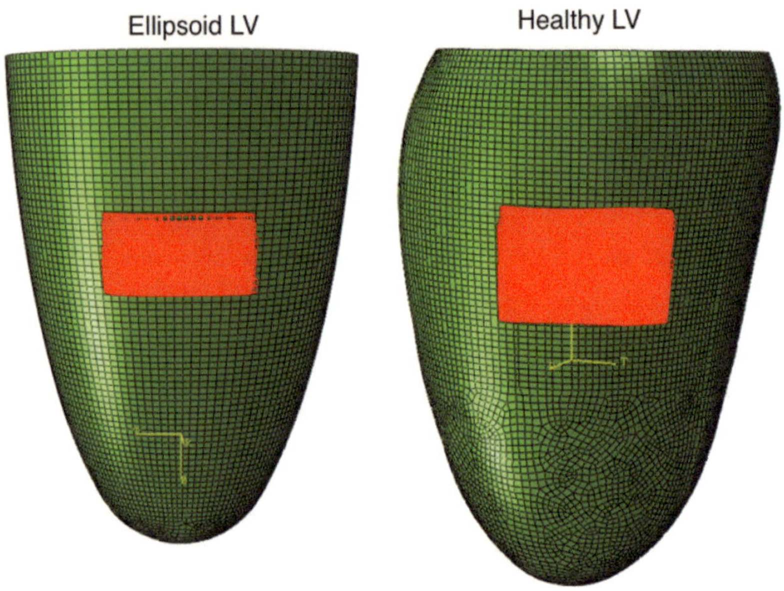

Figure 2. The synthetic acute ischemia generated on ellipsoid and healthy LV obtained from US images. The elements highlighted in red show the considered zone for zero active stress while other elements in green have a homogeneous active contraction value (160 kPa). Here, the systolic pressure was defined to be 11.24 kPa.

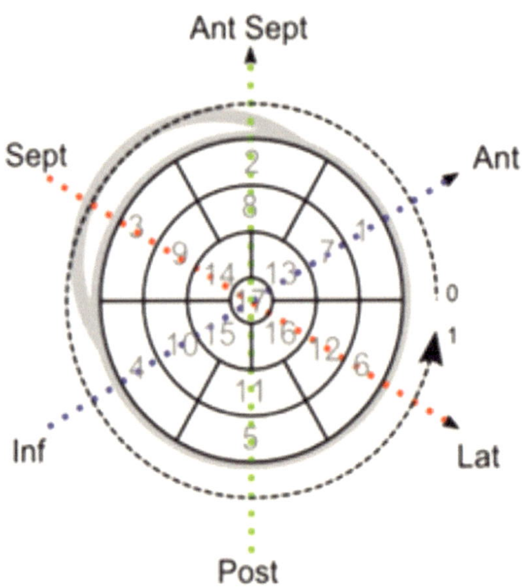

Figure 3. The AHA (American Heart Association) convention which describes the LV model in 17 regions. The study cases were divided into 4 separate regions as basal, mid-cavity, apical and apical cap. These regions were again split into several slices to build 17 regions. Copyrights reserved to GE Healthcare for this illustration of AHA regions.

2.2.2. *Healthy reference mesh*

The healthy mesh obtained from US imaging in Section 2.1 was used in this study case. The abnormal zone for this mesh was defined on the mid-cavity anterior wall (**Figure 2**). The boundary condition, systolic blood pressure, contraction model and the MPs were attributed as in the ellipsoid study case. The midwall regions were also generated in order to follow the regional deformations through the systolic phase. Reorientation of the fibre directions in abnormal LV tissue is an open question [31–34]. Therefore, we leave the fibres unchanged in the abnormal zone as defined for a healthy LV case in Section 2.1.

2.3. Prediction of abnormal tissue zone for LBBB patients

A cohort of patients suffering from LBBB was available for studying our proposed method for abnormal zone detection (with chronic infarcts). Left bundle branch block (LBBB) is a cardiac conduction abnormality which causes the LV to contract later than the right ventricle. We presented, previously, our FE method for a healthy LV contraction. In order to introduce the patient data to the FE software, we developed an in-house code to morph the reference FE mesh to the patient geometries. We demonstrated the steps for estimating homogeneous active contraction value data of acute ischemia in Section 2.2.

Eight LBBB patients were recruited after informed consent at Rikshospitalet, Oslo, Norway. LV triangulated mesh geometries were acquired by a standard GE Healthcare echocardiography examination [21]. The patient's LV cavity pressures were measured via an arterial catheter inside the left ventricle's cavity. The 17 regional strains were measured using 4D strain tracking EchoPac® US system manufactured by GE Healthcare [35]. EchoPac® algorithm calculates the classical longitudinal, circumferential and area strains for each segment at the midwall between endocardial and epicardial surfaces from the segment's dimensions [35] (**Figure 4**).

From area strain (*AS*), we can calculate the radial strain (*RS*) as detailed by Heimdal [35] from the incompressibility assumption (R = Volume/Area) of the cardiac tissue:

$$RS = -\frac{\frac{AS_{ES}-AS_{ED}}{AS_{ED}}}{\frac{AS_{ES}-AS_{ED}}{AS_{ED}+1}}. \tag{5}$$

We morphed the reference mesh (refer to Section 2.1) onto the geometry of each patient at ED time step for which US geometries were acquired. For this, endocardial and epicardial nodes of the deformable mesh were projected onto the patient's triangulated surfaces from a defined LV *centerline* [17] with rigid and non-rigid transformation methods employing an in-house developed Matlab® code. In order to deform the reference bulk model with intermediate nodes, we used FE elastic rigid body deformation employing the displacement vectors obtained from boundaries projection trajectories [17]. An in-house program coded in Matlab® found the closest nodes to the midwall mesh nodal positions obtained from the EchoPac® system for each patient at ED. Therefore, we can follow the evolution

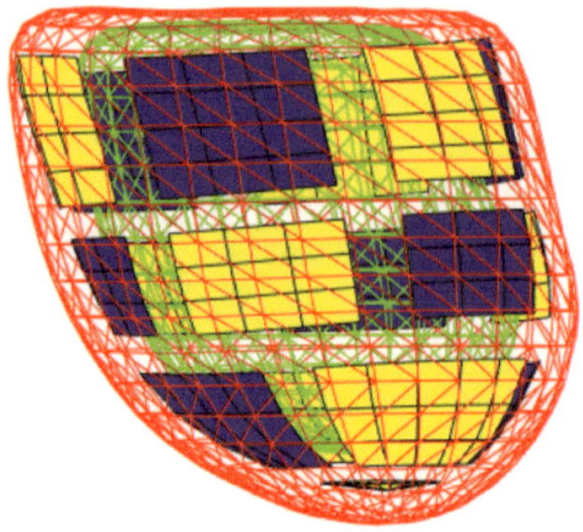

Figure 4. The midwall mesh example for a patient obtained from EchoPac®. The red and green triangles are the epicardium and endocardium surfaces, respectively. The yellow and purple meshes are segment's midwall mesh. These meshes permit us to follow the LV deformation through a cardiac cycle.

Case	**#1**	**#2**	**#3**	**#4**	**#5**	**#6**	**#7**	**#8**
ES pressure (kPa)	16.8	14	14.27	15.47	12.67	16.53	14.53	8666

Table 1. The ES pressure values for LBBB patients measured through aortic valves.

of LV during its systolic phase by calculating the deformations of each segment's mesh in area, radial circumferential and longitudinal strains.

For each patient, after application of the mesh morphing method, we employed the pressure values at ES from pressure curves obtained during the medical intervention (**Table 1**). This cavity pressure was applied as the boundary condition on the endocardial surface as previously mentioned in Section 2.1. For the sake of simulation costs, for each patient, we considered a set of a_f values from the literature starting at 60–280 kPa with 5 kPa of increments. Then, the LSQ simply takes the a_f which returns the minimum cost value.

3. Results

In this section, we describe the results of applying the proposed method to synthetic reference data and patient data from a group of LBBB patients.

3.1. Application to synthetic data

For the ellipsoid mesh, the closest match was achieved for a_f=155 kPa, which gave a cost function value of 0.0096. The EF for the reference ischemic case was 41.32% and the closest match was 43%. **Figure 5** shows the strains for the reference case (left) and the closest matching case with homogenous contraction (middle). The difference between the two is shown in the right panel, and demonstrates that the method identifies the correct location of the ischemic zone (starred).

Figure 6 shows the results of applying the method on the healthy LV geometry, with synthetically generated acute ischemic data. In this case, a minimum cost function value of 0.0387 was obtained for a_f=130 kPa. Strain values are shown for the reference ischemic case (left) and the closest matching case (middle), while the difference between the two (error) is shown on the right. We observe that the ischemic zone is easily detectable from the error plots.

3.2. Application on LBBB patients' data

We applied the mesh morphing method explained in Section 2.3 to construct patient-specific FE meshes for 8 LBBBB patients, shown in the figure by Behdadfar et al. [17]. **Table 2** shows

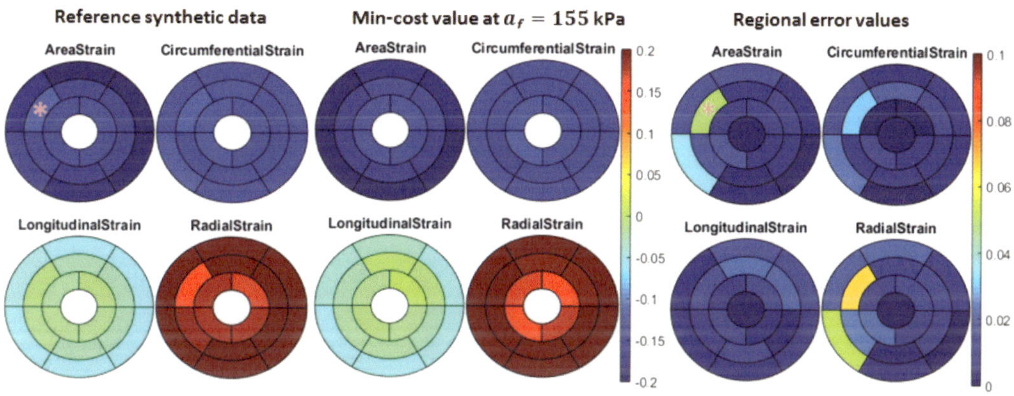

Figure 5. The regional deformations resulting from FE simulation and synthetic acute ischemia for the ellipsoid reference mesh based on AHA standards. The ellipsoid reference synthetic acute ischemia, the closest match for regional deformation as well as the error are presented in this figure. The algorithm has successfully detected the abnormal zone at mid-cavity (starred) as well as its impact on the neighboring tissue (Basal inferior).

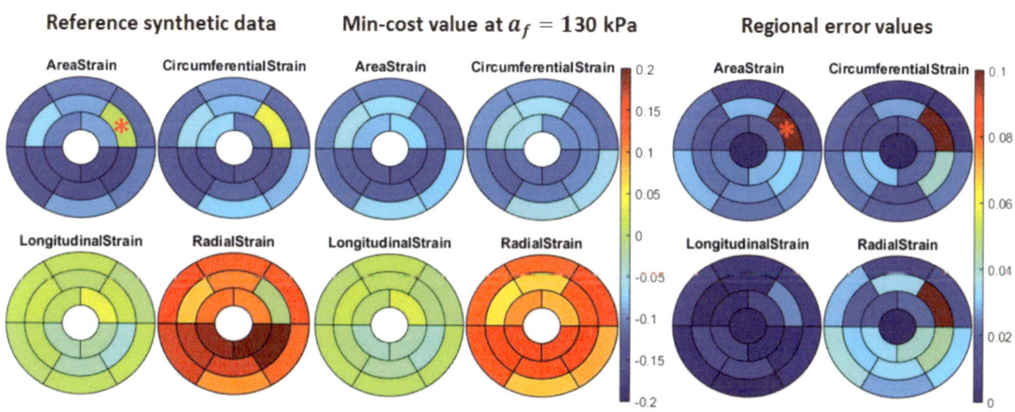

Figure 6. The healthy FE simulations and the regional deformation results based on AHA standards are shown in this figure. The results are presented for the reference generated acute ischemia, the closest match and the regional errors. The starred region is the actual generated zone with zero active stress value (mid-anterior wall).

the minimum cost value and the AAS values for each patient. In addition, the measured and simulated ED and ES cavity volumes are shown, as well as the EFs for both cases.

Case	*CostValue*	a_f (kPa)	EDV-S (ml)	ESV-S (ml)	EF-S%	EDV-P (ml)	ESV-P (ml)	EF-P%
#1	0.5279	130	160.764	139.827	13.02	171.3	121.8	28.72
#2	0.1960	135	196.815	140.20	28.76	215.9	159.4	26.16
#3	0.1298	135	179.602	161.53	10	179.3	131.3	26.77
#4	0.1686	95	120.082	124.195	Inflated	128.3	111.7	12.93
#5	—	—	—	—	—	319.1	241.2	24.41
#6	0.3358	180	168.118	132.808	21	179.7	111.2	38.11
#7	0.7901	175	242.429	273.670	Inflated	255.7	219.4	14.19
#8	0.1616	75	99.594	87.167	12.47	98.78	79.98	19

Table 2. The LBBB patients data measured (–P) and the FE results (–S). The ED volume (EDV), ES volume (ESV), LSQ cost value, optimized active stress (a_f) and EF are shown in this table. Patient 5 had convergence issues.

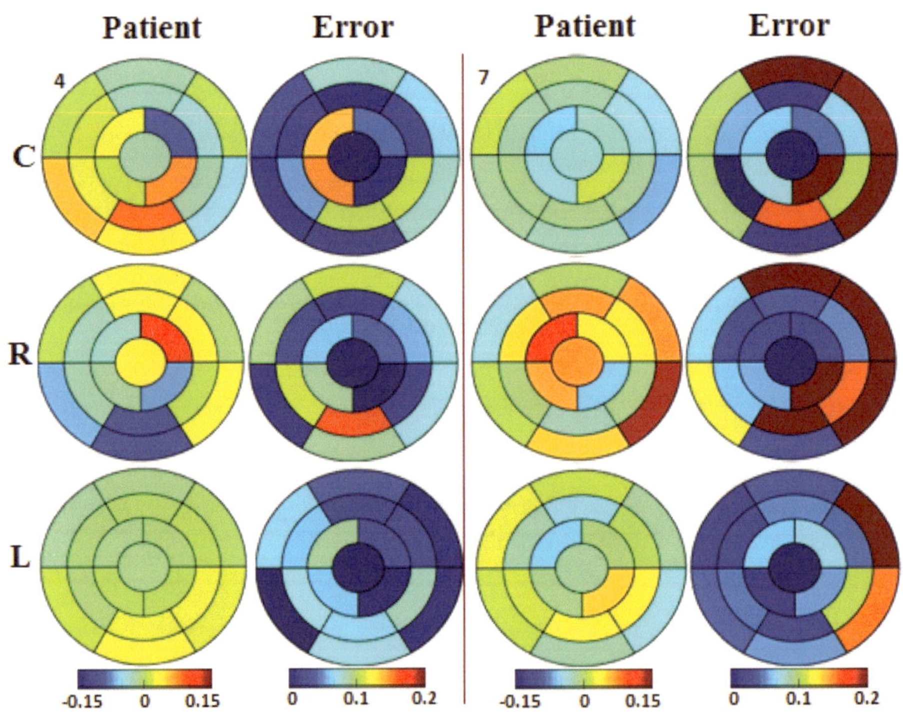

Figure 7. The LBBB patient's circumferential (C), radial (R) and longitudinal (L) strains at ES provided by EchoPac® US system of patients 4 and 7. The deformation differences between patient's data and the FE results from LSQ application under AHA standards are also shown. In this figure, we can observe that the maximum/minimum value (left column) of the 4-posterior, and 7-lateral regions are also the regions of maximum deviations observed in the FE results (right column), respectively.

The deformations obtained from US are in circumferential, longitudinal and area strain of the midwall mesh. Then, the RS was obtained by incompressibility hypothesis of the LV segments as explained by Heimdal [35]. The radial, circumferential and longitudinal strains are shown in **Figure 7** for patients 4 and 7 where the pipeline detected the abnormal zone. The FE strain results were subtracted from the patient's respective data and are shown in this figure as well.

Figure 8 shows the transversal and longitudinal cuts of LBBB patients' geometries superimposed by the FE simulation results for the optimal AAS. These cuts are tuned to show the maximum error zone (from 17 segments), obtained from LSQ application of regional deformation. Patient 5 had convergence issues and was not considered for further analysis.

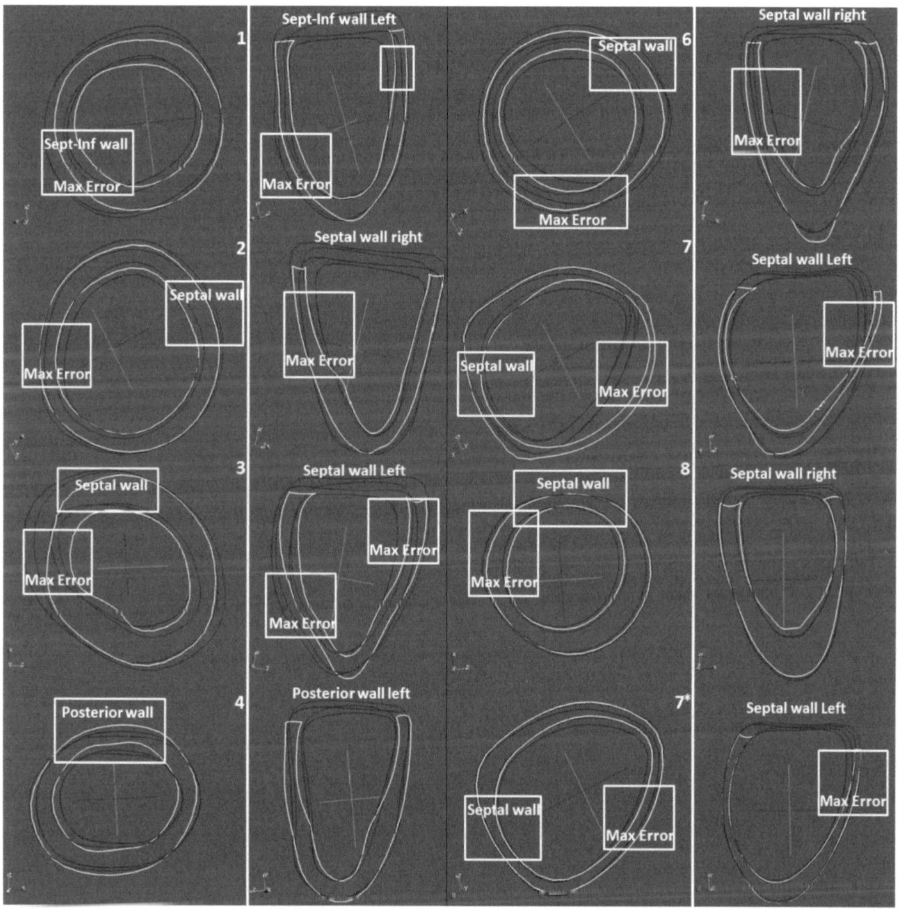

Figure 8. The transversal (first and third columns) and longitudinal (second and fourth columns) cuts of LBBB patient geometries (1–8) obtained from EchoPac® US system at ED (red lines) and ES (blue lines). The patient's data were superimposed with the FE simulation geometry for optimal AAS at ES (white lines). In this case, if the maximum error happened to be at the septal wall segment, the cut (longitudinal and transversal) passes through this segment in FE simulation and patient's geometry. The results for increasing MPs by 12 times are also shown here (7*). The patient 5 had no convergence success in this study.

4. Discussion

In this study, a new approach for detecting potentially infarcted areas was first validated on synthetic data and then applied to a cohort of 8 LBBB patients before resynchronization. The results revealed zones of moderate heterogeneities which were often of smaller thickness but the heterogeneities were significantly less pronounced than that revealed for a synthetic case of acute ischemia. The method also revealed that the tissue tends to be stiffer in the lateral wall of LBBB patients. It is very interesting to notice that the obtained results confirm what was already observed by other researchers using standard medical imaging. More specifically, Veress et al. [4] showed the typical septum-related abnormal wall motion and impairment of wall thickening during systole, which caused LV remodeling. Often, technologies such as MRI or PET (positron emission tomography) were used to characterize the infarct heterogeneities as well as histological images [36–38]. We examined if such ability to detect abnormal tissue can stand for novel 4D strain EchoPac® system.

In order to detect the abnormal tissue, we identified an AAS for all FE meshes which was the closest match to the patient's midwall mesh deformation (**Figure 1**). This AAS represents a homogeneous contraction for each patient [15, 16]. In this condition, it is expected that for a healthy and homogeneous contraction, the FE deformation responses will be different in abnormal tissue than the rest of the LV model. In addition, this value represents the average movement of remote (uninfarcted) and injured tissue.

Often, patients suffering from abnormal contractility are evaluated by an optimized gradient of activation stress map. Wenk et al. [39] have developed an animal-specific FE model for such reconstruction by minimizing the regional deformation error between experimental data and the FE model. In this study, a border zone was considered for early stage of tissue damaging process (due to calcium concentrations) which relates the injured to the remote tissue. They confirm that the infarct zone has no contractile action (zero active value).

4.1. Impact of MPs on the FE LV deformation

In **Table 2**, the AASs are mentioned for optimal cost values. These identified values are strongly coupled to the wall thickness, the blood pressure and the cavity volume. The FE results are based on the midwall strain deformation which is not representative data for the complete wall motion and might be affected by artifacts. Some meshes are inflated such as in cases 4 and 7 in **Table 2**, even if, these cases are the most successful results of the abnormal tissue detection. The reason for this inflation might be the compliance MPs for the studied cases. To study this hypothesis, we increased the elastic parameters (c_1 and c_2) by factors [2, 4, 5, 7, 9, 11] to analyze the behavior of the patient FE simulation to this increase in tissue rigidity.

For this test, patient 7 has been selected as the posterior and neighboring walls were deformed dramatically in FE simulation while these walls had not been moved during ED to ES movement. The cost value for this test from 0.7901 with 175 kPa of AAS was reduced to [0.1893, 0.0775, 0.0626, 0.0592, 0.0591, 0.0564], respectively, and it is shown in **Figure 4** for factor 12 (c_1 and c_2) in 7*. Novak et al. [40] showed that the aneurysmal wall is stiffer than the remote tissue as well. In this test, we observed that the results (7*) were improved by increasing the rigidity of the tissue MPs. It has been previously investigated, with a mathematical model and experimental tests, that the infarct tissue stiffen (despite dilated infarctions) [41]. However, the infarct tissue properties are still under investigation for various accompanying pathologies such as LBBB.

Figure 8 shows several successful zone detections wherein the maximum error happens to be at the abnormal region. In case 1, the maximum deformation was observed at the Inf-Sept-AntSept regions where this neighborhood wall slightly inflates (blue lines at Max-error in longitudinal cut) and the method detected this region successfully. However, in case 6, the inhomogeneous strain was observed at the septal wall wherein the method detected the posterior wall as the maximum error. These results show that the strain data in some cases can be difficult to be judged on the detected zone and is subjective to the visual detection of the patient's strain and geometry data. However, a FE simulation of pathology cases permit us to narrow down the potentially defeated zone to less regions, especially, in case 4 and 7 in **Figure 7** and to study the mechanical state of the cardiac tissue by analyzing the wall stress as a post-processing step.

The results showed a good agreement with several patient deformations in RS, which has been shown to be a better indicator than circumferential or longitudinal deformations due to the homogeneous distribution of these deformation values, for discrimination of possible heterogeneities in the active stress and abnormal tissue movement. We observed that the identified active stress is highly coupled to the patient geometry and wall thickness [42]. This is the advantage of the new generations of US system in extracting the RS from measuring the surface of a given segment that is not possible for modalities such as tagging MRI [43].

4.2. Remodeling in LBBB patients and its impact on the pipeline results

The LBBB, itself, causes tissue remodeling due to the redistribution of LV workload in the long run, especially, in circumferential shortening, cardiac mass, septal hypoperfusion and myocardial blood flow [44–47]. However, this pathology is, often, the result of other cardiac diseases. Statistically, 40% of patients with cardiomyopathy (CMP), weakening of the heart muscle and congestive heart failure have unsynchronized ventricular contraction. The resynchronization procedure helps in reverse remodeling and hospitalization-free survival rate of 70–90% in these patients [48–50].

The observed regional differences did not exist in the case of ellipsoid and healthy meshes illustrated previously, where the wall thickness is nearly homogeneous. Thus, the change in MPs or wall thickness in LBBB patients with previous infarct history should reduce the efficiency of this method for some patients with high heterogeneity in the wall deformation due to tissue remodeling. In **Figure 8** and **Table 2**, we can observe that the FE simulation responses in the maximal discrepancies with the patient's data are mostly over or under estimates of the tissue deformation. These maximal discrepancies have been observed to be at the high heterogeneities in wall thickness.

Patient 5 had convergence issues due to large cavity volume (319 ml at ED) and thin wall thickness (remodeled tissue). The large cavity volume is related to an aneurysmal bulging which made contraction simulation fail to reach a solution.

Several studies showed that LBBB patients respond poorly (30–50%) to resynchronization procedure for multiple reasons and cases with developed scarred tissue tend to not respond at all [51–53]. This study is a tool for patient cases which are not yet affected by this remodeling phase and are in the early stages of LBBB pathology. Information on areas with pathology within the left ventricular wall may be helpful in planning therapy with a resynchronization pacemaker [54].

4.3. Limitations

One major limitation in this study is the choice of material and contraction models to simplify the complexity and computational costs. In addition, we defined an a_f value which is also a brutal simplification for AAS identification procedure. However, with all this simplifications, the time of each simulation on a 12-core system was 72 h in average. One issue might be the small elements generated by developed mesh morphing procedure that reduced the time steps in the FE solver. One natural step can be improving the material model to anisotropic from the state-of-the-art [24]. The mesh morphing method should also be improved to reduce the computational costs in further work.

Another limitation is the lack of patient's history information. In this study, the patients were known to have LBBB pathology with infarct history but there was no other information on co-morbidities that may cause depressed myocardial contraction. The large cavity volume, low EF and low wall thickness can be related to various pathologies such as idiopathic dilated CMP, and ischemic cardiomyopathy. So in this work, it is not possible to categorize the patients with their pathologies (such as patient 5) and the identified AAS. We considered a stress-free configuration to simulate the systolic phase for our cohort so this issue should be further addressed.

5. Conclusion

In this study, a new approach for detecting potentially infarcted areas was introduced, validated and then applied onto a cohort of eight LBBB patients before their cardiac resynchronization therapy. The results revealed zones of moderate heterogeneities which were often of regions of thinner wall. However, the heterogeneities were significantly less pronounced than what was revealed for a synthetic case of acute ischemia, which we interpreted as an effect of remodeling induced by the therapy. The method also revealed that the tissue tends to be stiffer in the lateral wall of LBBB patients, as the deformations are not as pronounced as they are in the simulation. This study is promising for the assessment of LBBB and its quantification using FE simulations. Again, this illustrates the importance of patient-specific FE simulations in the domain of cardiac biomechanics.

Further work is required to transfer the promising synthetic results to real acute ischemic patient cases. A possible improvement is to reconstruct the patient fiber orientations from MRI imaging modalities such as diffusion tensor and tagging MRI to improve the deformation trajectories during contraction [55]. The possibility to compare this study results with cardiac MRI for identifying the abnormal tissue is also an interesting future step. Finally, it would be interesting to compare the reconstructions made with our methodology on LBBB patients at different stages of remodeling after the cardiac resynchronization treatment.

Acknowledgements

The authors gratefully acknowledge the support and data provided by the Center for Cardiological Innovation, funded by the Research Council of Norway. SA is grateful to the European Research Council for grant ERC-2014-CoG BIOLOCHANICS.

Author details

Sareh Behdadfar[1,2], Laurent Navarro[1,2], Joakim Sundnes[3,5], Molly Maleckar[4], Hans Henrik Odland[5] and Stephane Avril[1,2]*

*Address all correspondence to: avril@emse.fr

1 Mines Saint-Etienne, Saint Etienne, France

2 SaInBioSE, INSERM, U1059 and Université de Lyon, Saint Etienne, France

3 Simula Research Laboratory Oslo, Norway

4 The Allen Institute for Cell Science, Seattle, USA

5 Department of Cardiology, Center for Cardiological Innovation, Oslo University Hospital, Oslo, Norway

References

[1] Fishbein MC, Maclean D, Maroko PR. The histopathologic evolution of myocardial infarction. Chest. 1978;**73**(6):843-849

[2] Sabbah HN, Wang M, Gupta RC, Rastogi S, Ilsar I, Sabbah MS, Kohli S, Helgerson S, Lee RJ. Augmentation of left ventricular wall thickness with alginate hydrogel implants improves left ventricular function and prevents progressive remodeling in dogs with chronic heart failure. JACC: Heart Failure. 2013;**1**(3):252-258

[3] Lee LC, Wall ST, Klepach D, Ge L, Zhang Z, Lee RJ, Hinson A, Gorman JH, Gorman RC, Guccione JM. Algisyl-lvr-tm with coronary artery bypass grafting reduces left ventricular

wall stress and improves function in the failing human heart. International Journal of Cardiology. 2013;**168**(3):2022-2028

[4] Veress AI, Paul Segars W, Tsui BMW, Gullberg GT. Incorporation of a left ventricle finite element model defining infarction into the xcat imaging phantom. IEEE Transactions on Medical Imaging. 2011;**30**(4):915-927

[5] Sundnes J, Lines GT, Cai X, Nielsen BF, Mardal K-A, Tveito A. In: Computing the electrical activity in the heart. Vol. 1. Springer Science & Business Media; 2007

[6] Nejib Z. Theoretical and numerical study of the electric activity of the heart. Modeling and Numerical Simulation of Electrocardiograms [PhD thesis]. Université Paris Sud-Paris XI; 2009

[7] Shi WV, Chang TN, Zhou MC. Method to detect cardiac abnormalities based on electrocardiography and sinoatrial pacemaker model. In: 2010 International Conference on Mechatronics and Automation (ICMA), IEEE; 2010. pp. 566-571

[8] Oduneye SO, Pop M, Shurrab M, Biswas L, Ramanan V, Barry J, Crystal E, Wright GA. Distribution of abnormal potentials in chronic myocardial infarction using a real time magnetic resonance guided electrophysiology system. Journal of Cardiovascular Magnetic Resonance. 2015;**17**(1):1

[9] Underwood SR, Rees RS, Savage PE, Klipstein RH, Firmin DN, Fox KM, Poole-Wilson PA, Longmore DB. Assessment of regional left ventricular function by magnetic resonance. British Heart Journal. 1986;**56**(4):334-340

[10] Wael M, Ibrahim E-SH, Fahmy AS. Detection of cardiac function abnormality from mri images using normalized wall thickness temporal patterns. International Journal of Biomedical Imaging. 2016;**2016**

[11] Ibrahim E-SH. Myocardial tagging by cardiovascular magnetic resonance: Evolution of techniques–pulse sequences, analysis algorithms, and applications. Journal of Cardiovascular Magnetic Resonance. 2011;**13**(1):1

[12] Okrasinski SJ, Ramachandran B, Konofagou EE. Assessment of myocardial elastography performance in phantoms under combined physiologic motion configurations with preliminary in vivo feasibility. Physics in Medicine and Biology. 2012;**57**(17):5633

[13] Dandel M, Hetzer R. Echocardiographic strain and strain rate imaging clinical applications. International Journal of Cardiology. 2009;**132**(1):11-24

[14] Cerqueira MD, Weissman NJ, Dilsizian V, Jacobs AK, Kaul S, Laskey WK, Pennell DJ, Rumberger JA, Ryan T, Verani MS, et al. Standardized myocardial segmentation and nomenclature for tomographic imaging of the heart a statement for healthcare professionals from the cardiac imaging committee of the council on clinical cardiology of the american heart association. Circulation. 2002;**105**(4):539-542

[15] McVeigh ER, Prinzen FW, Wyman BT, Tsitlik JE, Halperin HR, Hunter WC. Imaging asynchronous mechanical activation of the paced heart with tagged MRI. Magnetic Resonance in Medicine. 1998;**39**(4):507-513

[16] Wyman BT, Hunter WC, Prinzen FW, McVeigh ER. Mapping propagation of mechanical activation in the paced heart with mri tagging. American Journal of Physiology-Heart and Circulatory Physiology. 1999;**276**(3):H881-H891

[17] Behdadfar S, Navarro L, Sundnes J, Maleckar M, Ross S, Odland HH, Avril S. A centerline based model morphing algorithm for patient-specific finite element modeling of the left ventricle. IEEE Transactions on Biomedical Engineering. 2017

[18] Hansegård J, Urheim S, Lunde K, Malm S, Rabben SI. Semiautomated quantification of left ventricular volumes and ejection fraction by real-time three-dimensional echocardiography. Cardiovascular Ultrasound. 2009;**7**(1):1

[19] Huyghe JM, Arts T, van Campen DH, Reneman RS. Porous medium finite element model of the beating left ventricle. American Journal of Physiology-Heart and Circulatory Physiology. 1992;**262**(4):H1256-H1267

[20] Bovendeerd PHM, Huyghe JM, Arts T, Van Campen DH, Reneman RS. Influence of endocardial-epicardial crossover of muscle fibers on left ventricular wall mechanics. Journal of Biomechanics. 1994;**27**(7):941-951

[21] Behdadfar S, Navarro L, Sundnes J, Maleckar MM, Avril S. Importance of material parameters and strain energy function on the wall stresses in the left ventricle. Computer Methods in Biomechanics and Biomedical Engineering. 2017;**20**(11):1223-1232

[22] Walker JC, Ratcliffe MB, Zhang P, Wallace AW, Fata B, Hsu EW, Saloner D, Guccione JM. Mri-based finite-element analysis of left ventricular aneurysm. American Journal of Physiology-Heart and Circulatory Physiology. 2005;**289**(2):H692-H700

[23] Dorri F, Niederer PF, Lunkenheimer PP. A finite element model of the human left ventricular systole. Computer Methods in Biomechanics and Biomedical Engineering. 2006;**9**(5): 319-341

[24] Holzapfel GA, Ogden RW. Constitutive modelling of passive myocardium: A structurally based framework for material characterization. Philosophical Transactions of the Royal Society of London A: Mathematical, Physical and Engineering Sciences. 2009;**367**(1902): 3445-3475

[25] Guccione JM, Costa KD, McCulloch AD. Finite element stress analysis of left ventricular mechanics in the beating dog heart. Journal of Biomechanics. 1995;**28**(10):1167-1177

[26] Usyk TP, Mazhari R, McCulloch AD. Effect of laminar orthotropic myofiber architecture on regional stress and strain in the canine left ventricle. Journal of Elasticity and the Physical Science of Solids. 2000;**61**(1–3):143-164

[27] Marchesseau S, Delingette H, Sermesant M, Ayache N. Fast parameter calibration of a cardiac electromechanical model from medical images based on the unscented transform. Biomechanics and Modeling in Mechanobiology. 2013;**12**(4):815-831

[28] McCulloch A, Waldman L, Rogers J, Guccione J. Large-scale finite element analysis of the beating heart. Critical Reviews in Biomedical Engineering. 1991;**20**(5–6):427-449

[29] Guccione JM, McCulloch AD. Mechanics of active contraction in cardiac muscle: Part I. Constitutive relations for fiber stress that describe deactivation. Journal of Biomechanical Engineering. 1993;**115**(1):72-81

[30] Hunter PJ, McCulloch AD, Ter Keurs HEDJ. Modelling the mechanical properties of cardiac muscle. Progress in Biophysics and Molecular Biology. 1998;**69**(2):289-331

[31] Holmes JW, Nunez JA, Covell JW. Functional implications of myocardial scar structure. American Journal of Physiology-Heart and Circulatory Physiology. 1997;**272**(5):H2123-H2130

[32] Holmes JW, Borg TK, Covell JW. Structure and mechanics of healing myocardial infarcts. Annu. Rev. Biomed. Eng. 2005;**7**:223-253

[33] Walker JC, Guccione JM, Jiang Y, Zhang P, Wallace AW, Hsu EW, Ratcliffe MB. Helical myofiber orientation after myocardial infarction and left ventricular surgical restoration in sheep. The Journal of Thoracic and Cardiovascular Surgery. 2005;**129**(2):382-390

[34] Chen J, Song S-K, Liu W, McLean M, Stacy Allen J, Tan J, Wickline SA, Xin Y. Remodeling of cardiac fiber structure after infarction in rats quantified with diffusion tensor MRI. American Journal of Physiology-Heart and Circulatory Physiology. 2003;**285**(3):H946-H954

[35] Heimdal A. 4d Strain: Advanced Research Application for Quantitative Echocardiography. GE Healthcare: United Kingdom; 2011

[36] Walker JC, Ratcliffe MB, Zhang P, Wallace AW, Hsu EW, Saloner DA, Guccione JM. Magnetic resonance imaging-based finite element stress analysis after linear repair of left ventricular aneurysm. The Journal of Thoracic and Cardiovascular Surgery. 2008;**135**(5):1094-1102

[37] Arevalo HJ, Vadakkumpadan F, Guallar E, Jebb A, Malamas P, Wu KC, Trayanova NA. Arrhythmia risk stratification of patients after myocardial infarction using personalized heart models. Nature Communications. 2016;**7**

[38] Pop M, Sermesant M, Mansi T, Crystal E, Detsky J, Yang Y, Fefer P, McVeigh ER, Dick A, Ayache N, et al. Characterization of post-infarct scars in a porcine model—A combined experimental and theoretical study. In: International Conference on Functional Imaging and Modeling of the Heart. Springer; 2009. pp. 1-10

[39] Wenk JF, Sun K, Zhang Z, Soleimani M, Ge L, Saloner D, Wallace AW, Ratcliffe MB, Guccione JM. Regional left ventricular myocardial contractility and stress in a finite element model of posterobasal myocardial infarction. Journal of Biomechanical Engineering. 2011;**133**(4):044501

[40] Novak VP, Yin FCP, Humphrey JD. Regional mechanical properties of passive myocardium. Journal of Biomechanics. 1994;**27**(4):403-412

[41] Kelley ST, Malekan R, Gorman JH, Jackson BM, Gorman RC, Suzuki Y, Plappert T, Bogen DK, Martin G, Sutton SJ, Henry Edmunds L. Restraining infarct expansion preserves left

ventricular geometry and function after acute anteroapical infarction. Circulation. 1999; **99**(1):135-142

[42] Götte MJW, van Rossum AC, Twisk JWR, Kuijer JPA, Tim Marcus J, Visser CA. Quantification of regional contractile function after infarction: Strain analysis superior to wall thickening analysis in discriminating infarct from remote myocardium. Journal of the American College of Cardiology. 2001;**37**(3):808-817

[43] Denney TS, Gerber BL, Yan L. Unsupervised reconstruction of a three-dimensional left ventricular strain from parallel tagged cardiac images. Magnetic Resonance in Medicine. 2003;**49**(4):743-754

[44] Kasai T, Gordon DePuey E, Shah AA. Decreased septal wall thickening in patients with left bundle branch block. Journal of Nuclear Cardiology. 2004;**11**(1):32-37

[45] Mahrholdt H, Zhydkov A, Hager S, Meinhardt G, Vogelsberg H, Wagner A, Sechtem U. Left ventricular wall motion abnormalities as well as reduced wall thickness can cause false positive results of routine spect perfusion imaging for detection of myocardial infarction. European Heart Journal. 2005;**26**(20):2127-2135

[46] Sugihara H, Tamaki N, Nozawa M, Ohmura T, et al. Septal perfusion and wall thickening in patients with left bundle branch block assessed by technetium-99m-sestamibi gated tomography. The. Journal of Nuclear Medicine. 1997;**38**(4):545

[47] Vernooy K, Verbeek XAAM, Peschar M, Crijns HJGM, Arts T, Cornelussen RNM, Prinzen FW. Left bundle branch block induces ventricular remodelling and functional septalhypoperfusion. European Heart Journal. 2005;**26**(1):91-98

[48] Prinzen FW, Cheriex EC, Delhaas T, van Oosterhout MFM, Arts T, Wellens HJJ, Reneman RS. Asymmetric thickness of the left ventricular wall resulting from asynchronous electric activation: A study in dogs with ventricular pacing and in patients with left bundle branch block. American Heart Journal. 1995;**130**(5):1045-1053

[49] Breithardt O-A, Stellbrink C, Herbots L, Claus P, Sinha AM, Bijnens B, Hanrath P, Sutherland GR. Cardiac resynchronization therapy can reverse abnormal myocardial strain distribution in patients with heart failure and left bundle branch block. Journal of the American College of Cardiology. 2003;**42**(3):486-494

[50] Ypenburg C, van Bommel RJ, Jan Willem Borleffs C, Bleeker GB, Boersma E, Schalij MJ, Bax JJ. Long-term prognosis after cardiac resynchronization therapy is related to the extent of left ventricular reverse remodeling at midterm follow-up. Journal of the American College of Cardiology. 2009;**53**(6):483-490

[51] Auricchio A, Stellbrink C, Sack S, Block M, Vogt J, Bakker P, Huth C, Schöndube F, Wolfhard U, Böcker D, et al. Long-term clinical effect of hemodynamically optimized cardiac resynchronization therapy in patients with heart failure and ventricular conduction delay. Journal of the American College of Cardiology. 2002;**39**(12):2026-2033

[52] Abraham WT, Fisher WG, Smith AL, Delurgio DB, Leon AR, Loh E, Kocovic DZ, Packer M, Clavell AL, Hayes DL, et al. Cardiac resynchronization in chronic heart failure. New England Journal of Medicine. 2002;**346**(24):1845-1853

[53] Kerckhoffs RCP, McCulloch AD, Omens JH, Mulligan LJ. Effects of biventricular pacing and scar size in a computational model of the failing heart with left bundle branch block. Medical Image Analysis. 2009;**13**(2):362-369

[54] Constantino J, Hu Y, Trayanova NA. A computational approach to understanding the cardiac electromechanical activation sequence in the normal and failing heart, with translation to the clinical practice of crt. Progress in Biophysics and Molecular Biology. 2012;**110**(2):372-379

[55] Ming-Ting W, Tseng W-YI, Su M-YM, Liu C-P, Chiou K-R, Wedeen VJ, Reese TG, Yang C-F. Diffusion tensor magnetic resonance imaging mapping the fiber architecture remodeling in human myocardium after infarction correlation with viability and wall motion. Circulation. 2006;**114**(10):1036-1045

Chapter 6

Non-Conventional Radiotherapy for Total Body Irradiation: Antecedents, Current Research and Perspectives

Francisco Mesa-Linares

Additional information is available at the end of the chapter

http://dx.doi.org/10.5772/intechopen.73026

Abstract

In addition to the conventional techniques used in radiotherapy, certain procedures, special-called for the treatment of both some cancer diseases and clinical application are usually required. Such practices typically manifest a technical problem with respect to the equipment used, which requires important adjusts that diverge significantly from the standard implemented in the common treatments. Total body irradiation is one of those special techniques, in which the radiation target is the entire patient body. In a broad sense, the concept covers all radiation processes with photon beam fields more wide than standard field size. Treatment with total body irradiation is usually applied with purpose of providing immunosuppression to prevent rejection in bone marrow transplantation procedure. Diseases such as aplastic anemia and a varied number of leukemia and lymphomas respond favorably to this treatment scheme. Beams of megavoltage photons, such as Cobalt sources and linear accelerators, are used for such purposes. In this chapter, the technique will be studied analyzing its definition and first applications. The chapter includes a description of the main treatment schemes on which it is based, covering the calibration process, ergonomic criteria as well as the main contributions in the clinical research field, opportunity fields and novel research perspectives.

Keywords: total body irradiation, radiotherapy, lineal accelerator, non-conventional, in vivo dosimetry, portal imaging, ergonomics

1. Introduction

Radiotherapy, surgery and chemotherapy are the three main modalities used in oncology for the treatment of diseases caused by malignant cells [1, 2]. Unlike other medical specialties, which essentially maintain their sureness in the clinical knowledge and experience of the medical specialist, in radiotherapy, due to the use of ionizing radiations, it is required besides the confidence in modern technologies, as well as the nearest collaboration of many other professionals. The radiotherapy team consists of a group of oncologists, medical physicists, dosimetrists, nurses and technicians [3], all with different levels of training, but with a goal, the need to understand the physical basis of radiation therapy.

Radiotherapy is a specialized discipline in the field of medicine, which involves the use of high-energy ionizing radiation for the treatment of cancer cells [4]. The radiation sources used in this clinical field can be located throughout internally to the patients (brachytherapy) or external way (teletherapy). During the first 50 years of radiotherapy, technological progress was relatively scarce and based mainly on X-ray tubes, Van de Graaff generators and Betatrons. The invention of the Cobalt 60 machine [5] around 1950 by Harold Elford Johns in Canada, gave a new twist to the radiotherapy technique, becoming for several decades the most important tool for cancer treatments (**Figure 1**).

However, the most widely used system for radiotherapy treatments today is the use of Linear Accelerators (Linac). The concurrent development of this system overshadowed the extraordinary impact of the 60Co source, becoming the most widely used radiation source in modern radiotherapy.

Conventional radiotherapy is usually focused on traditional studies (breast cancer, cervical cancer, etc.) where the equipment is calibrated (**Figure 2**) for radiation beam emission with remote settings of 1.00 m and maximum radiation fields of 0.40 × 0.40 m [6, 7].

In addition to these conventional techniques, several procedures, special-called, for the treatment of certain diseases and clinical applications are required. Such procedures manifest a technical problem in essence because the equipment used requires certain modifications that diverge significantly from the adjustments implemented in the more common treatments. Total body irradiation (TBI) is one of those special techniques, in which the radiation target is the entire patient body. In a broad sense, the TBI concept covers all radiation processes with

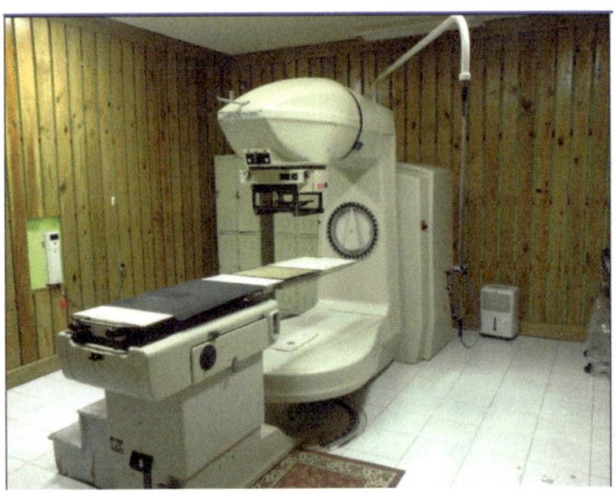

Figure 1. 60Co clinical unit (Theratronics, Ottawa, Canada). Courtesy of Ing. Antonio Almonte, from Dr. Heriberto Pieter Cancer Center, Santo Domingo, Dominican Republic.

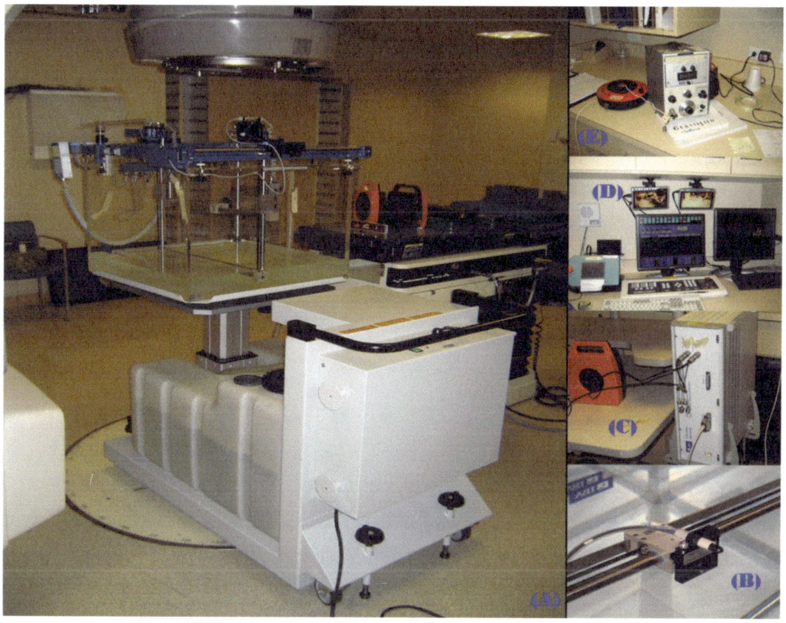

Figure 2. Varian linear accelerator for clinical use, and the basic equipment for radiotherapy calibrations. (A) Computerized water phantom system, (B) PTW ionization chamber N31003 no. 975; (C) Scanditronix Wellhofer; (D) Fixed computer system; and (E) Keithly CNMC electrometer. Courtesy of Dr. Carlos Esquivel, from Cancer Therapy & Research Center, San Antonio, Texas, USA.

long radiation fields, that is, with fields larger than the standard maximum of 0.40 m × 0.40 m. Megavoltage photon beams, such as Cobalt-60 sources and linear accelerators, are used for such purposes.

2. Total body irradiation

TBI is a technique accepted as radiotherapy treatment and frequently used in combination with chemotherapy as a complementary regimen for bone marrow transplants [8, 9]. Diseases such as aplastic anemia [10] and a varied number of leukemia and lymphomas [11, 12] respond to the TBI treatment. Ewing's sarcoma, advanced non-Hodgkin lymphomas, lung cancer and lymphosarcoma have also been treated in combination with TBI therapy [13].

The first applications of TBI date back to the early twentieth century, when in 1907 the German Friedrich Dessauer published the first work that has been recorded [14]. Another of the pioneering works on TBI, carried out in the United States, corresponds to the studies done by Heublein [15], who implemented an arrangement in which four patients could be irradiated simultaneously using a Coolidge tube.

A large number of authors have worked on the implementation of different arrangements for TBI applications, being probably the irradiation technique that considers the beam of radiation in a fixed position and keeps the patient in vertical position, the most commonly used by different cancer centers. However, the experimental results usually show significant variations in the dose levels between patients, which represent a poor reproducibility of the different protocols. These discrepancies may be influenced, to some degree, by illness and patient fatigue associated with chemotherapy sessions, which makes it difficult for many patients to remain in the proper treatment position during prolonged exposure times.

Many of the first clinical experiences with TBI were carried out in centers with special designs and facilities. However, and due to the increased need to treat an important variety of diseases, patients are now commonly treated in commercial units.

2.1. Treatment schemes for TBI

Basically, the TBI treatments fall inside two general categories: bilateral irradiation (lateral TBI) and antero-postero total body irradiation (AP-PA TBI). At the first one [16], patient is collocated up treatment bed, so the radiation beam is perpendicularly to the sagittal patient plane (**Figure 3**). In AP-PA TBI [17], on the other hand, the patient is placed in an anatomical position, either maintained vertically or installed in some arrangement designed so that the radiation beam is perpendicular to the patient coronal plane (**Figure 4**). In both cases, the patients are positioned in such a way that it can be completely covered by the area of the projected field. For what usually require the patient collaboration, such as asking the patient to bend their knees, in order to adequately cover the projected field.

TBI is normally implemented with the aim of achieving a homogeneous distribution of the dose at the level of the patient's median plane. However, the parameters such as the irregularities and thicknesses of the areas of the patient's contours to be irradiated have dimensions much greater than those observed in any other radiotherapy treatment therapy. Such considerations

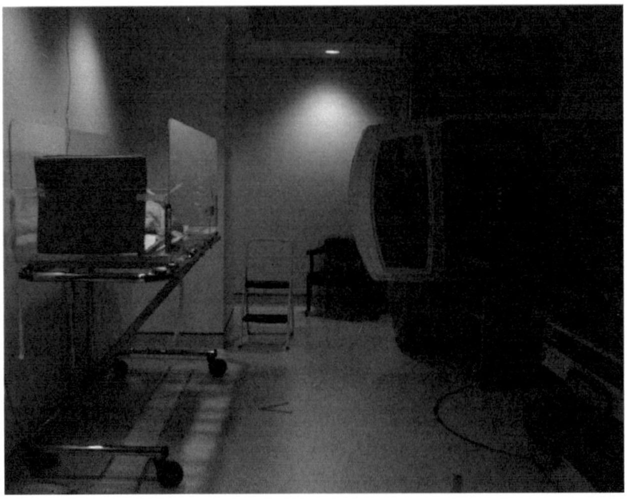

Figure 3. Image taken during one of the treatment sessions for lateral TBI at the Cancer Therapy & Research Center, San Antonio, Texas, USA. Image taken by Francisco Mesa.

http://dx.doi.org/10.5772/intechopen.73026

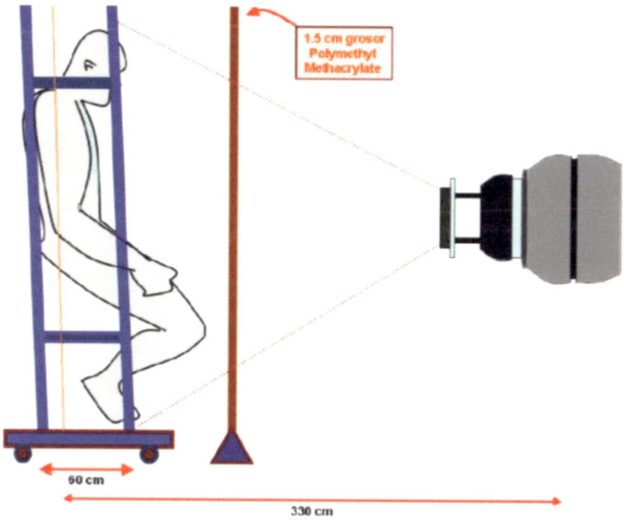

Figure 4. Illustrative diagram of the positioning of the patient during the implementation of the treatment. A vertical platform 0.015 m thick acrylic (polymethylmethacrylate) is placed in front of the patient to increase the skin dose.

seem to be more widely observable during the treatments of Lateral TBI, where in addition, the armoring technique of critical organs, such as the lung, does not turn out to be as efficient in practice as in the case of applications in AP-PA TBI.

The implementation of compensating filters is one of the most important procedures used in TBI for the correction of heterogeneity in the distribution of the dose. The arrangement formed by several sheets of lead of different thicknesses (**Figure 5**) allows the attenuation of the dose levels supplied, so that for a specific amount of *Monitor Unit* (MU) applied, different dose levels can be registered in the different contours of the body, in order to achieve the same distribution of the dose at the level of the patient's median plane. The considerable reduction of the dose levels with respect to the *build-up zone* (space or depth between the surface and the point of maximum ionization, and which is characteristic of each energy and type of radiation) is another factor to be considered regarding of the TBI applications. Such a reduction entails the application of percentages of much lower doses in skin, than the percentages in the rest of the body.

2.2. Dosimetric calibrations for TBI

The basic dosimetric parameters for TBI are the same as for standard radiotherapy, including dose rate, *percentage depth dose* (PDD), *tissue-maximum ratio* (TMR) and beam profiles (**Table 1**). However, these parameters must be measured under the specific conditions of TBI in order to obtain relevant data for clinical use (**Figure 6**). Many dosimetric problems related to the use of phantom and also radiation detectors should be considered for this type of non-conventional applications. In contrast to standard radiotherapy, for example, water phantoms are generally smaller than the field sizes and also smaller than the patient's dimensions. This causes different dispersion conditions that can generate adverse beam effects.

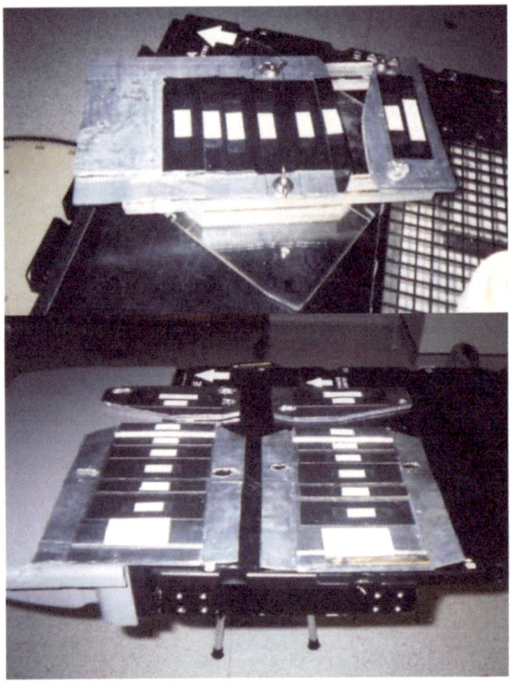

Figure 5. Design of the attenuation filters used to generate a homogeneous dose distribution at the level of the patient's median plane. Filter arrangements was calculated and designed to the contour of each patient. Courtesy of Cancer Therapy & Research Center, S.A., TX.

Basically, the material, equipment and general instrumentation for TBI consists of a lineal accelerator (i.e. Varian, Siemens, etc.) for clinical use; a solid water phantom (i.e. PMMA, RW3,); ionizing chambers (i.e. FC65-P Scanditronix Wellhöfer Farmer FC65/IC69; CC13 P-CC13–510-001 02); the Scanditronix Wellhofer (Farmer Scanditronix Wellhofer); a fixed basic computer system; a Keithly CNMC electrometer; a portal X-ray equipment for lateral or AP-PA linac-portal radiographs; a 1.2-cm acrylic beam spoiler and tray at the head of the gantry and thermoluminescent dosimeters for in vivo dose verification.

The determination of the type of energy used for the applications of TBI is a factor of high importance and depends on many dosimetric factors and clinical criteria.

The photon beams used for TBI have essentially the following properties: (a) point of maximum ionization is below the surface, registering, for example, for the energies of 6–18 MV, at depths of 0.018–0.032 m in water (**Figure 6**); (b) when is higher energy of the radiation beam, the lower the percentage of the dose is recorded on the surface; (c) photons have a high penetration power, registering dose levels of approximately 0.20–0.30 m deep with similar values to the surface, for energies of 6–18 MV, respectively; (d) below the *"build-up"* zone (maximum ionization), the PDD have greater intensity in photons of 18 MV than of 6 MV (**Figure 7**).

When reviewing the literature, a wider use consideration of energies of 6 MV of photons for TBI treatments is observed. However, a broader and more detailed discussion about the need and criteria of using one or another type of energy is necessary.

Dosimetric parameters	Conventional radiotherapy	Total body irradiation
Field size	≤0.40 m × 0.40 m	>1.20 m
Patient treatment distance	1.00 m	>3.00 m
Dose rate	0.05 Gy/s	0.00166–0.025 Gy/s
Dose per section	1.50 Gy/session	1.00 Gy/session
Total dose	40–50 Gy	12 Gy
Treatment technique	Source-surface distance/isocentric	Isocentric
Radiation source	Cobalt 60/lineal accelerator	Cobalt 60/lineal accelerator
Additional equipment	No	Compensation filters/special treatment bed
Calibration phantom	Computerized water phantom system	Solid phantom
Radiation detectors	PTW ionization chamber; Scanditronix Wellhofer; fixed computer system; Keithly CNMC electrometer	PTW ionization chamber; Scanditronix Wellhofer; fixed computer system; Keithly CNMC electrometer
In vivo dosimetry	No	Yes
Number of sections	1 dairy/20–40 day	2 dairy/3 day.

Table 1. Comparisons between the different dosimetric parameters that intervene in the both conventional treatment process and TBI. Description: Gy = Gray.

2.3. Treatment planning

The treatment planning stage (simulation) consists of location and identification of the area of the body to be irradiated, as well as the definition and recording of the geometric conditions and physical parameters related to the patient placement and installation. For the Lateral TBI scheme, patients are placed on the treatment bed, placed in the supine position with the knees

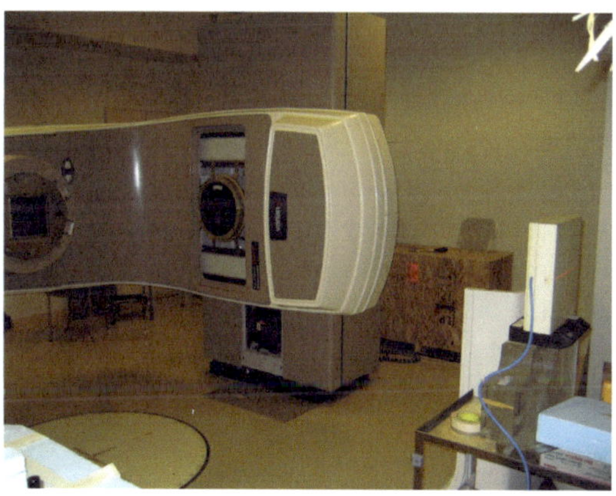

Figure 6. Experimental set-up for TBI calibration with a linear accelerator at the treatment distance (3.50 m), and an ionization chamber installed inside the PMMA solid phantom. Calibration process conduced at the Cancer Therapy & Research Center, San Antonio, Texas, USA. Courtesy of Dr. Carlos Esquivel, from Cancer Therapy & Research Center, San Antonio, Texas, USA.

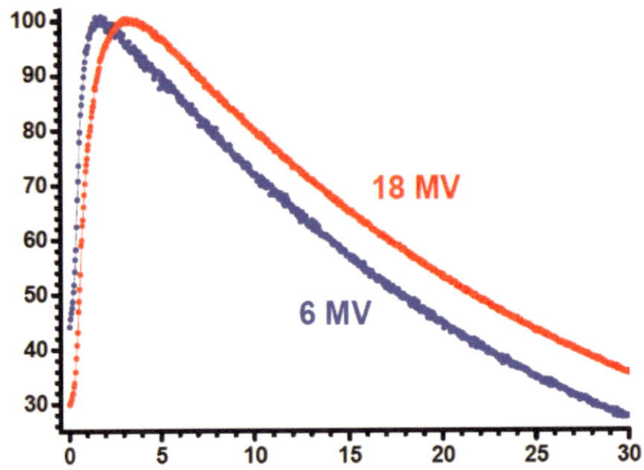

Figure 7. Behavior of the PDD for 6–18 MV photon beams, obtained with a Clinac 21EX linear accelerator, at the medical unit of high specialty, Mexican Institute of Social Security, form León, Guanajuato, Mexico.

in flexion, and placing the hands together on the abdomen. The arms in this position can serve as partial shielding of the lungs.

In the case of AP-PA TBI, for other hand, patient is placed in a kneeling chair position (**Figure 4**), and it is supported with its hands through handlebars set, holding in the chest by means of a holding strap, which keeps it in a fixed and stable position throughout the entire process. The assembly is installed inside an arrangement formed by stainless steel bars placed on a mobile base, occupying a space of 0.80 × 0.50 × 2.00 m. The system includes several cushions for the head, back and knee, in order to keep it in a comfortable position during the treatment sessions. In each case, dosimetrist must make sure that the patient is placed in a position that is comfortable and placed in such a way that it is completely localized in the projected radiation field. The contours of anatomical regions of interest (**Table 2**) are marked with permanent ink during this stage of the process. The regions of interest are usually identified in the head, neck, shoulders, breasts, abdomen, hips, thighs, knee and ankle.

The measurement of the greater thickness contour, the distance of the patient's surface area, the compensations (offset), the depth (thicknesses) of the contours (right–left, left–right, anterior–posterior, posterior–anterior), and all geometric parameter measurements were recorded at this stage of the procedure. Geometrical projections on the Gantry head, with respect to the different contours previously selected, in order to calculate the dimensions of the arrangement of sheets used for the design of the compensating filters, are determined. Subsequently, a radiographic plate of the lung is taken, which is used as a reference for the design of the protective lung blocks (**Figure 8**). For the treatment application, patients are usually cited a week after being subjected to the simulation process, and they are placed in a similar way to that process. Patients are placed inside a prismatic square box (for Lateral TBI) or stainless steel bars assembly (for AP-PA TBI). For the last one, 0.015 m thick acrylic (*polymethylmethacrylate*) vertical platform in front of the patient in order to increase the skin dose, was installed (**Figure 4**).

The system is installed at a suitable *source-axis distance* (SAD), with respect to the median plane, and in such a way that it is completely located in the field projected by the light output of the lin-

Anatomic contours	Anatomic localization descriptions	
	Lateral TBI	AP-PA TBI
Head	Along the longitudinal axis of the skull at the level of the pituitary fossa	Reference point defined along the longitudinal axis of the skull
Neck	Reference point defined along the patient's longitudinal axis at the level of C3/C4	It is not usually included
Shoulder	This reference point is defined as just inferior to the lateral 1/3 of the clavicle	Shoulders, lower zone 1/3 of lateral distance of clavicle
Chest	Along the patient's longitudinal axis at the level of the angle of Louis	Midline at the level of the sternum head
Abdomen	This reference point is defined as the point along longitudinal axis midplane at the level of the umbilicus	Point along navel level
Hip	Defined along the patient's longitudinal axis at the center of the pelvis at a level that is 1.0 cm superior to the symphysis pubis	Proximal femur at the level of the major trochanter
Thigh	It is not usually included	Mean distance between the ends of the femur
Knee	Along the midline in the midplane of the knee at the level of the middle of the patella	Knee, at the level of the middle of the kneecap
Ankle	Defined along the middle of the ankle at the level of the lateral malleolus	Tibia-fibula intersection

Table 2. Anatomical description of contours and location of points for dosimeter installation during dose verification for both lateral TBI and AP-PA TBI.

ear accelerator head. Once the patient is installed in the treatment position, the lead attenuation filters are placed and aligned to them so that their projections coincide with the contour marks of the anatomical regions indicated in the simulation process.

2.4. In vivo dose verification

In vivo dose verification are usually developed during the first treatment sessions with TLD-100 dosimeters previously characterized.

The TLD-100 is probably the best known dosimeter and the most widely used for clinical applications [18–23]. It was developed by J. R. Cameron in 1968 [24]. Chemically, it is composed of lithium fluoride doped with magnesium and titanium impurities (LiF, Mg, Ti). Widely accepted and commercially used, the TLD-100 is basically presented in the form of chips, with dimensions of 0.0032 m × 0.0032 m × 0.0009 m. They allow dose measurements between 10^{-6} and 1 Gy, in the linear response range; they present a high precision for measurements registration (from 1 to 2%); having 2640 kg/m^3 of density and an effective atomic number equal to 8.2, close to the biological tissue.

The dosimeters are placed at specific points of interest located in each contour defined in the simulation process (**Table 2**). They are installed on the skin of the patient under a few pieces

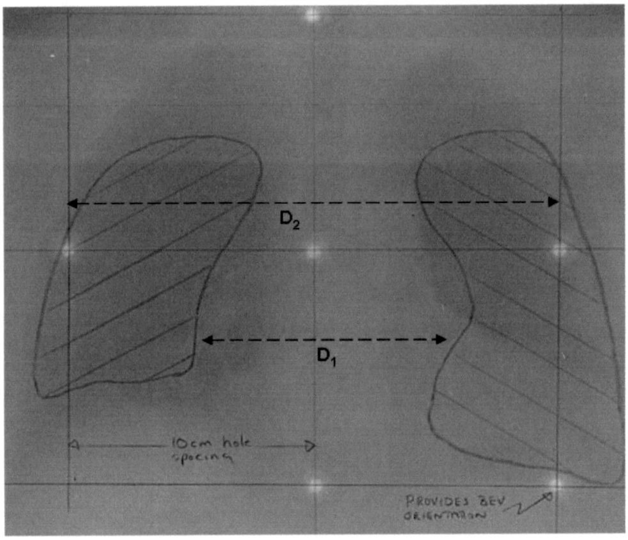

Figure 8. Lung radiography used for design of protective lung blocks. The distances from the medial plane to the medial side of the lung (*D* 1/2) and the lateral side of the lung (*D* 2/2) are shown.

(bolus) of tissue-equivalent material, to produce the maximum 0.015 m dose (*build-up*) in each reading. The dose verification at the level of the median plane is calculated for each contour by:

$$D_{Midplan} = \frac{L_{TLD}(nC) \times CF_{TLD}(^{cGy}/_{nC})}{ISL \times TMR} \tag{1}$$

where L_{TLD} is the raw thermoluminescence reading; CF_{TLD} is the calibration factor for TLD; *ISL* is the *inverse-square factor* and *TMR* is the *tissue-maximum ratio.*

2.4.1. Other in vivo dose detectors

Although thermoluminescent dosimeters are the most widely used detector for in vivo dose verification in total body irradiation, the development and implementation of new methods to determine dose levels during treatment sessions has been increasing. The use of Gafchromic EBT films [25–27], EDP-30 diodes [28] and other semiconductors [29] has been considered as an important alternative to achieve a more accurate and timely in vivo dosimetry.

However, the need to develop detectors for in vivo dosimetry that determine dose levels in a real time sense during the application of unconventional radiotherapy treatment continues to be an open opportunity for the scientific community.

3. Opportunity fields and novel research perspectives

Total Body Irradiation is a complex treatment modality that requires careful planning to specify the homogeneity in the dose distribution, as well as the location of the organs that will receive a reduced dose, or that must be completely shielded from the radiation beam.

Even though in general terms, aspects associated with the planning of radiation treatment have a scientific and methodological support regulated by international organizations through reports and recommendations [6, 7], it should also be considered that these regulations are essentially based on protocols associated on conventional radiotherapy. Regulations about the calibration processes based on the use of solid phantom and specific dosimetric settings for treatment distances greater than the standard (0.40 m × 0.40 m) are necessary for the strengthening of the technique. Similarly, the need to provide more evidence on the evolution of the tumor and its behavior in the face of the effect of radiation is evident [30]. Other criteria associated with the evaluation of different physical, biological, environmental and even perception variables could have a significant impact on the evolution of patients' health status.

The identification of anthropometric parameters, which are usually performed only during the first stage in treatment planning, and associated with certain very specific protocols, could provide relevant information regarding early recovery in patients with chronic diseases. In this sense, when reviewing the literature, it is clear the need to develop research works that provide more accurate information about the adequacy homogeneity in the distribution of doses during treatment sessions, as well as the location of organs that will receive a reduced dose or that must be "shielded" completely with respect to the radiation beam.

It is also observed the need to design ergonomic mechanisms that guarantee greater stability and comfort of the patients during the considerable treatment times. Together with the need for calculation and calibration systems with greater precision and accuracy, as well as the performing of in vivo dosimetry with greater reproducibility during treatment, constitute important opportunity areas for TBI.

4. Conclusions

De conventional radiotherapy concept, usually focused on traditional studies where the equipment is calibrated for radiation beam emission with remote settings of 100 cm and a maximum radiation fields of 0.40 m × 0.40 m, and is differences respect to TBI, as a non-conventional treatment scheme, was described. The TBI protocol has been carried out following the recommendations on clinical dosimetry calibrations of the TG-51 report [6], as well as the recommendations regarding the physical aspects of total body radiation provided by TG-29 [31]; last one published at 1986, what motivates the need to promote studies for its update according to the development of new technologies.

The protocol presented includes the development and description of the calculation process to determine both the dimensions and thicknesses of the dose compensation filters used to obtain a homogeneous dose distribution at the level of the patient's median plane. It also includes the development of thermoluminescent dosimetry for the verification of in vivo doses during the first sessions of treatment. The protocol was presented in two modalities: Lateral TBI and AP-PA TBI. In the first modality, the patients were placed on a treatment table, in supine position, with the knees bent upwards, inside a square prismatic box constructed of acrylic, and in such a way that they were completely inscribed in the projected field. In the second one, however, the patients were positioned within an arrangement designed for such purposes, where they were seated, adopting a kneeling chair position, and irradiated in AP and PA fields during each treatment session.

Basically both treatments have been made to be applied under the same medical prescriptions; however, the use of one or the other tends to depend essentially on the anthropomorphic characteristics, body type (size, size), and the type of cancer and stage of the cancer presented by the patients, as well as on the degree of precision desired of a certain specific part of the body.

When observing the experimental results of both techniques, obtained during the in vivo dose verification process, better levels of precision are observed with respect to the values registered for the Lateral TBI technique, which promotes, from this point of view, greater reliability regarding the other technique. It is also more convenient to apply this technique, when it is required to install the patient in a position of greater comfort, either by the state of fatigue or by the degree of disease that it presents. Treatments in AP-PA, conversely, are more convenient to perform when a more homogeneous dose distribution is desired at the level of the whole body. While the lung protection system adequately reduces the dose at the level of the lung, it is also true that this reduction affects a body area of greater area, thus generating a reduction in dose levels with respect to the different contours adjacent.

On the other hand, the AP-PA technique is also suitable for patients with greater body proportions such as: anthropometry, height, diameter, because they have a better location within the projected radiation field, as well as in obese patients, where a significant part of your chest or abdomen could result in a definition of a greater degree of irregularity in the corresponding contour, with respect to the other contours of the body.

It is important to note that both arrangements were implemented using the same facilities of a conventional radiotherapy treatment room, which is important mainly because it facilitates the implementation of both protocols in any standard radiotherapy unit.

The chapter covered the basic dosimetric parameters for TBI, calibration process and it comparison with respect to the standard radiotherapy adjusts. A description about the in vivo dose verification system with thermoluminescent dosimetry and other detector used was discussed, as well as the need to develop detectors for in vivo dosimetry that determine dose levels in a real time sense during the application of unconventional radiotherapy treatment was presented.

Finally a description about important opportunities field, future discussions and novel research perspectives were summarized.

Acknowledgements

The author wish to recognize contributions of the Cancer Therapy & Research Center staff, for images, orientation, facilities and all collaboration in this project. Many special thanks to Doctors Niko Papanikolaou, Tony Y. Eng and Carlos Esquivel for their invaluable advice and academic guidance, as well as for the great opportunity to develop research at CTRC, USA. Also, they are grateful to the Modesto Sosa, PhD and the General Secretary and the Academic Interchanges Direction and Inter-Institutional Relations of the Guanajuato University, at México, for their support. The report has been inspired as part of the upcoming collaboration of the Technological University Paso del Norte with both the Medical Center of High Specialty and the Regional Institute of Cancer Treatment at Ciudad Juarez, represented by Dr. Emilio Torres-Medina and Dr. Elías Abbud-Abbud, respectively. All clinical and experimental activities were partially supported for Autonomous University of Santo Domingo, at Dominican Republic.

Conflict of interest

The authors declare the absence of any conflict of interest associated with this report. It will be a pleasure to be able to attend any observations that will be required.

Author details

Francisco Mesa-Linares

Address all correspondence to: fmesa@uabc.edu.mx

School of Engineering and Technology Sciences ECITEC, Autonomous University of Baja California, Tijuana, Baja California, Mexico

References

[1] Baskar R, Lee KA, Yeo R, Yeoh KW. Cancer and radiation therapy: Current advances and future directions. International Journal of Medical Sciences. 2012;**9**(3):193-199. DOI: 10.7150/ijms.3635

[2] Lee JH, Barich F, Karnell LH, Robinson RA, Zhen WK, Gantz BJ, Hoffman HT. National Cancer Data Base report on malignant paragangliomas of the head and neck. Cancer. 2002;**94**(3):730-737. DOI: 10.1002/cncr.10252

[3] Fraass B, Doppke K, Hunt M, Kutcher G, Starkschall G, Stern R, Van Dyke J. American association of physicists in medicine radiation therapy committee task group 53: Quality assurance for clinical radiotherapy treatment planning. Medical Physics. 1998; **25**(10):1773-1829. DOI: 10.1118/1.598373

[4] Widder J. The origins of radiotherapy: Discovery of biological effects of X-rays by Freund in 1897, Kienböck's crucial experiments in 1900, and still it is the dose. Radiotherapy and Oncology. 2014;**112**:150-152. DOI: 10.1016/j.radonc.2014.06.010

[5] Cameron J. A new kind of ray: The radiological sciences in Canada. Aldrich JE, Lentle BC, editors. Medical Physics. 1996:1-435. DOI: 10.1118/1.597806

[6] Almond PR, Biggs PJ, Coursey BM, Hanson WF, Huq MS, Nath R, Rogers DW. AAPM's TG-51 protocol for clinical reference dosimetry of high-energy photon and electron beams. Medical Physics. 1999;**26**(9):1847-1870. DOI: 10.1118/1.598691

[7] Andreo P, Burns DT, Hohlfield K, Huq MS, Kanai T, Laitano F, Smyth V, Vynckier S. Absorbed dose determination in external beam radiotherapy, an international code of practice for dosimetry based on standards of absorbed dose to water. Technical Report Series No. 398. Vienna: International Atomic Energy Agency; 2000

[8] Cao N, Ford E, Nyflot M, et al. TBI technique improvements for anesthetized pediatric patients based on near-miss incident reporting. International Journal of Medical Physics, Clinical Engineering and Radiation Oncology. 2016;**5**(4):270-280. DOI: 10.4236/ijmpcero.2016.54027

[9] Al-Malki MM, Castillo JJ, Sloan JM, Re A. Hematopoietic cell transplantation for plasmablastic lymphoma: A review. Biology of Blood and Marrow Transplantation. 2014;**20**(1):1877-1884. DOI: 10.1016/j.bbmt.2014.06.009

[10] Kim H, Lee KH, Kim I, Sohn SK, Jung CW, Joo YD, Kim SH, Kim BS, Choi JH, Kwak JY, et al. Allogeneic hematopoietic cell transplantation without total body irradiation from unrelated donor in adult patients with idiopathic aplastic anemia: Fludarabine versus cyclophosphamide-ATG. Leukemia Research. 2014;**38**:730-736. DOI: DOI.org/10.1016/J.LEUKRES.2014.01.002

[11] Hoster E, Geisler CH, Doorduijn J, Van del Holt B, Walewski J, Bloehdorn J, et al. Total body irradiation after high-dose cytarabine in mantle cell lymphoma: A comparison of Nordic MCL2, HOVON-45, and European MCL younger trials. Leukemia. 2016;**30**:1428-1430. DOI: 10.1038/leu.2015.322

[12] Block AM, Silva SR, Welsh JS. Low-dose total body irradiation: An overlooked cancer immunotherapy technique. Journal of Radiation Oncology. 2017;**6**(2):109-115. DOI: 10.1007/s13566-017-0303-x

[13] Minard-Colin V, Brugieres L, Reiter A, et al. Non-Hodgkin lymphoma in children and adolescents: Progress through effective collaboration, current knowledge, and challenges ahead. Journal of Clinical Oncology. 2015;**33**(27):2963-2974. DOI: 10.1200/JCO.2014.59.5827

[14] Dessauer FA. New design for radiotherapy. Archives of Physical Medicine. 1907;**2**(1):218-223

[15] Heublein AC. Preliminary report on continuous irradiation of the entire body. Radiology. 1932;**18**:1051-1062. DOI: 10.1148/18.6.1051

[16] Mesa F, Eng T, Fuller C, Esquivel C, Papanikolaou N, Sosa M. Implementation of a lateral total body irradiation technique with 6 MV photons. Journal of Radiotherapy in Practice. 2011;**10**:45-54. https://doi.org/10.1017/S1460396910000221

[17] Mesa F, Papanikolaou N, Esquivel C, Eng T, Fuller C, Sosa M. Prescribed and measured dose differences for an AP-PA TBI protocol with compensation filter and ergonomic patient support. Journal of Medical Imaging and Radiation Sciences. 2017;**48**(3):301-306. DOI: 10.1016/J.JMIR.2017.06.001

[18] Ducha MA, Ginjaumea M, Chakkora H, Ortegaa X, Jornetb N, Ribasb M. Thermoluminescence dosimetry applied to in vivo dose measurements for total body irradiation techniques. Radiotherapy and Oncology. 1998;**47**(3):319-314. DOI: 10.1016/S0167-8140(98)00013-9

[19] Palkoskava P, Hlavata H, Dvorak P, Novotny J, Novotny J. In vivo thermoluminescence dosimetry for total body irradiation. Radiation Protection Dosimetry. 2002;**101**(1-4):597-600. DOI: 10.1093/oxfordjournals.rpd.a006058

[20] Barquero R, Mendez R, Iñiguez MP, Vega HR, Voytchev M. Thermoluminescence measurements of neutron dose around a medical linac. Radiation Protection Dosimetry. 2002;**101**(1-4):493-496. DOI: 10.1093/oxfordjournals.rpd.a006035

[21] Waligorski MPR. What can solid state detectors do for clinical dosimetry in modern radiotherapy? Radiation Protection Dosimetry. 1999;**85**(1):361-366. DOI: 10.1093/oxfordjournals.rpd.a032872

[22] Pradhan AS. Thermoluminescence dosimetry and its applications. Radiation Protection Dosimetry. 1981;**1**(3):153-167. DOI: 10.1093/oxfordjournals.rpd.a079971

[23] Kron T. Applications of thermoluminescence dosimetry in medicine. Radiation Protection Dosimetry. 1999;**85**(1):333-340. DOI: 10.1093

[24] Cameron JR, Suntharalingam N, Kenney GN. Thermoluminescent Dosimetry. Madison: University of Wisconsin Press; 1968

[25] FC S, Shi C, Papanikolaou N. Clinical application of GAFCHROMIC® EBT film for in vivodose measurements of total body irradiation radiotherapy. Applied Radiation and Isotopes. 2008;**66**(3):389-394. DOI: 10.1016/j.apradiso.2007.09.015

[26] Andres C, del Castillo A, Tortosa R, Alonso D, Barquero R. A comprehensive study of the Gafchromic EBT2 radiochromic film. A comparison with EBT. Medical Physics. 2010;**37**(12):6271-6278. DOI: 10.1118/1.3512792

[27] Rah JE, Hwang UJ, Jeong H, Lee SY, Lee DH, Shin DH, Yoon M, Lee SB, Lee R, Park SY. Clinical application of glass dosimeter for in vivo dose measurements of total body irradiation treatment technique. Radiation Measurements. 2011;**46**:40-45. DOI: 10.1016/j.radmeas.2010.08.013

[28] Jornet N, Ribas M, Eudaldo T. Calibration of semiconductor detectors for dose assessment in total body irradiation. Radiotherapy and Oncology. 1996;**38**:247-251. DOI: 10.1016/0167-8140(95)01677-5

[29] Ramm U, Licher J, Moog J, Scherf C, Kara E, Bottcher D, Rodel C, Mose S. In vivo dosimetry with semiconducting diodes for dose verification in total-body irradiation. Strahlentherapie und Onkologie. 2008;**184**:376-380. DOI: 10.1007/s00066-008-1823-5

[30] Mi H, Petitjean C, Dubray B, Vera P, Ruan S. Prediction of lung tumor evolution during radiotherapy in individual patients with PET. IEEE Transactions on Medical Imaging. 2014;**33**(4):995-1003. DOI: 10.1109/TMI.2014.2301892

[31] Van Dyk J, Galvin JM, Glasgow GP, Podgorsak EB. The physical aspects of total and half body photon irradiation. A report of Task Group 29, Radiation Therapy Committee, American Association of Physicists in Medicine. Report No. 17. New York; 1986. p. 60. Available from: https://www.aapm.org/pubs/reports/RPT_17.pdf

Chapter 7

Automatic Image Analysis and Recognition for Ultrasound Diagnosis and Treatment in Cardiac, Obstetrics and Radiology

Zisheng Li, Peifei Zhu, Takashi Toyomura and Yoshimi Noguchi

Additional information is available at the end of the chapter

http://dx.doi.org/10.5772/intechopen.76284

Abstract

Ultrasound image analysis and recognition techniques for improving workflow in diagnosis and treatment are introduced. Fully automatic techniques for applications of cardiac plane extraction, foetal weight measurement and ultrasound-CT image registration for liver surgery navigation are included. For standard plane extraction in 3D cardiac ultrasound, multiple cardiac landmarks defined in ultrasound cardiac examination guidelines are detected and localized by a Hough-forest-based detector, and by six standard cardiac planes, cardiac diagnosis is extracted following the guideline. For automatic foetal weight measurement, biparietal diameter (BPD), femur length (FL) and abdominal circumference (AC) are estimated by segmenting corresponding organs and regions from foetal ultrasound images. For ultrasound-CT liver image registration, initial alignment is obtained by localizing a corresponding portal vein branch from an intra-operative ultrasound and preoperative CT image pair. Then portal vein regions of the ultrasound-CT image pair are extracted by a machine learning method and are used for image registration.

Keywords: ultrasound image analysis, automatic measurement, machine learning, image registration

1. Introduction

Ultrasound imaging is widely used for examination and navigation in diagnosis and therapy procedures. However, ultrasound image quality is affected by speckle noise and physical characteristics of the patient. Moreover, ultrasound image acquisition highly depends on skills and experience of a user. As a result, high-accuracy measurement or navigation by using ultrasound imaging is difficult and time-consuming. Therefore, it is necessary to develop automatic ultrasound image analysis and recognition techniques to improve the efficiency and accuracy in workflow of diagnosis and treatment. In this chapter, automatic techniques for applications of cardiac plane extraction [1], foetal weight measurement and ultrasound-CT image registration for liver surgery navigation [2, 3] are introduced.

2. Standard plane extraction in 3D cardiac ultrasound

2.1. Overview of standard plane extraction

Cardiac ultrasound device is a necessary tool that can help clinicians evaluate, diagnose and treat cardiac diseases. In a routine cardiac examination, six standard planes, apical four chamber (A4C), apical two chamber (A2C), apical three chamber (A3C), parasternal short-axis mitral valve (PSX MV), parasternal short-axis papillary muscle (PSX PM) and parasternal short-axis apex (PSX AP) [4] are commonly used to evaluate the structure and function of the heart. However, diagnosis using ultrasound device still suffers from inefficiency problems, such as user/patient dependency and complex operational procedures. There are market needs of improving the workflow in ultrasound diagnosis. According to such needs, there is a trend that cardiac diagnosis is changing from 2D diagnosis to 3D diagnosis. In conventional 2D ultrasound diagnosis shown in **Figure 1(a)**, 1D array probe is used for data acquisition. Clinicians have to change multiple positions to check different views of the heart. As a result, a large number of images are acquired. During the measurement, clinicians have to evaluate and diagnose cardiac diseases manually, which is inefficient. On the other hand, in 3D ultrasound diagnosis in the near future shown in **Figure 1(b)**, a 2D array probe is used to acquire a whole heart volume. Measurement then can be applied automatically using the acquired volume, and it is much more efficient than the conventional 2D ultrasound diagnosis. Therefore, an efficient and robust method for automatic plane extraction in 3D cardiac ultrasound is significant for improving the cardiac examination workflow.

There are literatures on automatic detection and localization in medical volume data [5–8]. However, large computational load is required since the standard planes were extracted in an independent way in most of these works. This chapter introduces a machine learning framework based on the cardiac-ultrasound examination guideline presented by the American Society of Echocardiography [4]. The presented framework is shown in **Figure 2**. The procedures are as follows: (1) Feature point detection: The above guideline indicates that clinicians should firstly localize the A4C plane with image features of mitral annulus and apical in the examination. Accordingly, three anatomical points on the A4C plane are selected as targets of localization, and a Hough forest classifier [9, 10] is modified and applied for the feature point localization. As a result, the A4C plane is localized. (2) Plane initialization: The guideline indicates that there are anatomical regularities between A4C and the other five planes. Therefore, initial locations of the other five planes are estimated by using that of the A4C plane and

http://dx.doi.org/10.5772/intechopen.76284

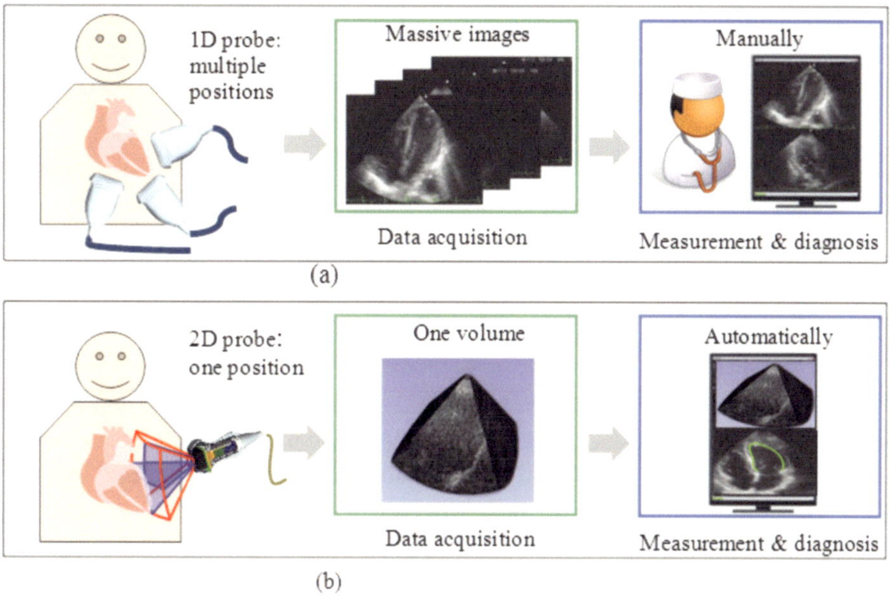

Figure 1. (a) Conventional 2D ultrasound diagnosis and (b) 3D ultrasound diagnosis in the future.

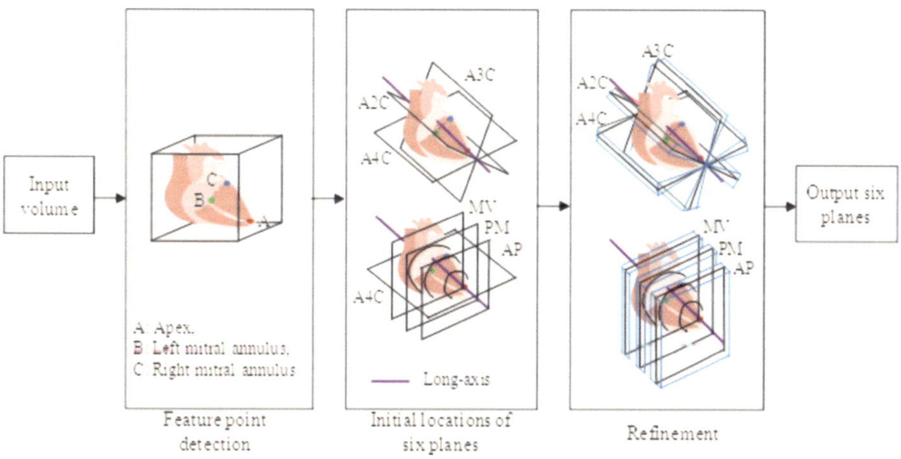

Figure 2. Framework of guideline-based machine learning for standard plane extraction.

the anatomical regularities. (3) Plane refinement: Plane location refinement is required due to individual differences. Here, a regression forest method with locations constraints is presented for the plane localization refinement.

2.2. Standard plane initialization

In the presented method, three anatomical points, including the apex, left mitral annulus (left MA) and right mitral annulus (right MA), are selected for the localization of the A4C plane. Feature point localization is performed by utilizing a Hough forest classifier, which is presented in Section 2.2.1. Moreover, on the purpose of improving the accuracy and speed, a multi-scale hierarchical searching approach is presented in Section 2.2.2. Next, initial locations of all six planes are determined by using the locations of the earlier feature points and anatomical regularities. The explanation is given in Section 2.2.3.

2.2.1. Hough forest

A Hough forest classifier is modified and applied for feature point localization. This approach can map from image patches to anatomical locations. In our work, Hough forest is extended from 2D to 3D by using 3D image features and 3D Hough voting.

Training process: In Hough forest, each tree T is constructed on the basis of a set of image patches $P_i = (I_i, c_i, d_i)$, where I_i is image appearance of the image patch in 3D, c_i is class label (positive or negative) and d_i is the offset from the patch location centre to the target location centre. For a background patch, d_i is undefined. When the training converges, each image patch reaches a leaf node L of the constructed tree. The information of such patches is stored in the leaf node. Such information includes C_L, which is the proportion between the object patches, the background patches and $D_L = \{d_i\}$ which is the list of the offset vectors. During training, before reaching the leaf node, each patch goes through binary tests of non-leaf nodes in each tree. The binary test is based on the appearance vector (image feature vector) of each patch $I_i = (I_i^1, I_i^2, \ldots, I_i^N)$ where I_i^n refers to one channel of the feature vector, such as pixel intensity, first or second derivative and so on. During training, each node needs to be constructed with a binary test. A key point of Hough forest is how binary test is evaluated. In order to achieve an optimal test, the uncertainties in both the class labels and the offset vectors should decrease towards the leaves. Class label uncertainty $U_1(A)$ and offset uncertainty $U_2(A)$ are defined as:

$$U_1(A) = -|A| \cdot \sum p(c|A) \ln(p(c|A)), \tag{1}$$

$$U_2(A) = \sum_i (\mathbf{d}_i - \mathbf{d}_A)^2, \quad when \ c_i = 1, \tag{2}$$

where A is a set of patches, $|A|$ is the number of patches, $p(c|A)$ is the proportion of patches with label c in set A and d_A is the mean offset vector over all object patches. The node construction process is as follows [10]. Given a training set of patches, we firstly generate a pool of pixel tests $\{t^k\}$ by uniformly choosing one feature channel and two pixel locations inside a patch. The threshold τ for each test is chosen randomly from the range of differences observed on the data. Then, the randomized decision is made whether the node should minimize the class label uncertainty or the offset uncertainty. The process can be represented as:

$$\arg\min_{\mu}\left(U_*(\{P_i | t^k = 0\}) + U_*(\{P_i | t^k = 1\})\right), \tag{3}$$

where * indicates the uncertainty measure for the node (U_1 or U_2), $\{P_i | t^k = 0\}$ is the set of patches that satisfy the binary test $t^k = 0$ and $\{P_i | t^k = 1\}$ is the set of patches that satisfy the binary test $t^k = 1$.

Testing process: The detection process can be divided into regression and voting steps. The regression process is as follows. Step 1: for each pixel at a location p, an image patch surrounding the pixel with a fixed size is extracted and input is fed to the trained forest (trees). Step 2: when passing through each node, the patch is split into either the left or the right child node according to the binary test of the trained node. All pixels in the image are going through the forest simultaneously in steps 1–2 until they reach the leaves. During the voting process, the information stored in the leaves is used to cast the probabilistic Hough votes to the location of the object centre. Leaf information consists of proportion C_L and offset vectors D_L, so that C_L/D_L is defined as a weight value for a vote. Each pixel with its location p votes to all locations $\{p-d \mid d \in D_L\}$ (the candidate positions of the object centre) with a weight value C_L/D_L. After Gaussian filtering of all the accumulated votes at all the candidate positions from each pixel, a Hough image $V(x)$ can be obtained. The maxima position of the Hough image can be considered as the detected object centre, that is, the detected vessel branch.

2.2.2. *Coarse-to-fine localization strategy*

In order to improve the efficiency and accuracy of the landmark localization, a coarse-to-fine strategy is applied to both the training and test procedures. In the training procedure, images of training data are firstly down-sampled to a low resolution level and the corresponding Hough forest classifiers are trained. Then regions of interest (ROIs) centred at the landmark locations are extracted for the training of the fine resolution level. In the test (detection) procedure, the rough landmark location is estimated at the coarse level and the ROI centred at the detected location are extracted at the fine resolution level. By applying the fine-level classifiers, final detection result can be achieved.

2.2.3. *Plane initialization with anatomical regularity*

First, the A4C plane can be localized by the detection of the three feature points. The cardiac long axis can also be localized by point A and the centre of point B and point C, as shown in **Figure 2**. Next, the A3C and A2C planes can be localized by rotating the A4C plane along the long axis at angles of 53 degrees and 129 degrees, respectively. Finally, localization of the three short axis planes (MV, PM and AP) starts from positions that are perpendicular to A4C. Then they can be localized by translating along the long axis with proportional intervals of 1/6, 3/6 and 5/6.

2.3. Plane refinement with regression forest

The refinement is divided into two parts: refinement of the long-axis planes and refinement of the short-axis planes. The long-axis planes include A4C, A3C and A2C. Because the location of A4C can be determined by three detected points, only the refinement of the other two long-axis planes (A3C and A2C) is considered. According to the guideline of standard plane extraction, the long-axis planes should all pass through the long axis. An example of plane A3C is shown in **Figure 3**. A geometry theorem defines that two lines (not collinear) will uniquely determine a plane. Therefore, the long-axis planes can be localized by the long-axis and an angle around the long axis α. Here, the angle α equals to a line with a point intersected at the long axis. Since the long axis is fixed by the detected feature points, during refinement, only

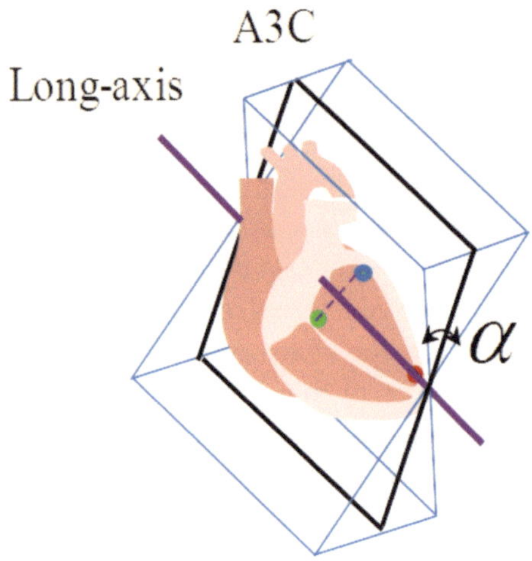

Figure 3. An example of long-axis plane refinement.

the angle α of the planes (A3C and A2C) needs to be optimized. A method based on regression forest [7, 8] is used for searching the optimized angles.

According to the guideline of standard plane extraction, the short-axis planes should be perpendicular to the long axis. An example of plane PM is shown in **Figure 4(a)**. In addition, there is a geometry theorem defining that a plane is uniquely determined by a nonzero normal vector and a point. Therefore, the short-axis planes can be localized by the long axis (nonzero normal vector) and a point on each plane. Here, anatomical feature points are selected on each plane for refinement, as shown in **Figure 4(b)**. Three points selected as feature points are (1) for plane MV, the centre of mitral valve (marked as point D), (2) for plane PM, centre of papillary muscle (the bottom one, marked as point E) and (3) for plane AP, the centre of apex (marked as point F). Point D, E and F are first detected from the 3D volume for the refinement of the short-axis planes. Each short-axis plane is then determined by the long axis and each detected point. The detection of point D, E and F also uses the method which is presented in Section 2.2.1. However, for the feature points on the short axis, only coarse-level detection is

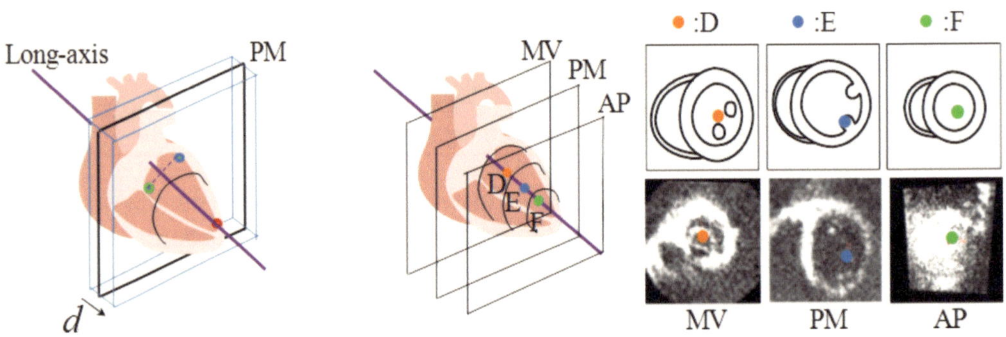

Figure 4. An example of long-axis plane refinement. (a) Short-axis plane refinement and (b) three anatomical feature points on short-axis planes.

applied. Evaluation experiments demonstrated that the fine-level detection applied for these points led to a larger error. This is mainly because these three points are lacking of discriminative local features which are crucial for the success of the fine-level detection. Therefore, the whole volume of information of the heart is applied to predict the final location of the three feature points on the short-axis planes.

2.4. Experiments and discussions

The presented method was evaluated on a 3D cardiac ultrasound dataset that was available in the works of Tobon-Gomez et al. [11]. The database includes 15 datasets from healthy volunteers. Only the end diastole frame from each volunteer is used in this experiment. A fivefold cross-validation scheme was performed in the evaluation. Moreover, data augmentation was performed by randomly rotating and scaling the original cardiac volume. As a result, 120 volumes were generated for training, and 30 volumes were generated for evaluation in each of the fivefold validations. Dimensions of the volumes were around 320 × 347 × 241, and image resolution is 0.5 × 0.5 × 0.5 mm^3.

To measure the accuracy of plane extraction, that is, how close the extracted plane is from the ground-truth plane, two evaluation standards were presented by Lu et al. [5]. Such standards are angle error and distance error. The angle error is defined as the angle between the

	Angle (degree)	Distance (mm)	Run time (s)
MSL [5]	11.3 ± 8.0	3.7 ± 2.1	2
Class-specific RF [7]	6.4 ± 4.3	4.2 ± 3.8	30
Proposed method	8.3 ± 4.9	2.7 ± 2.3	0.8

Table 1. Comparison of point detection between Hough forest and proposed method.

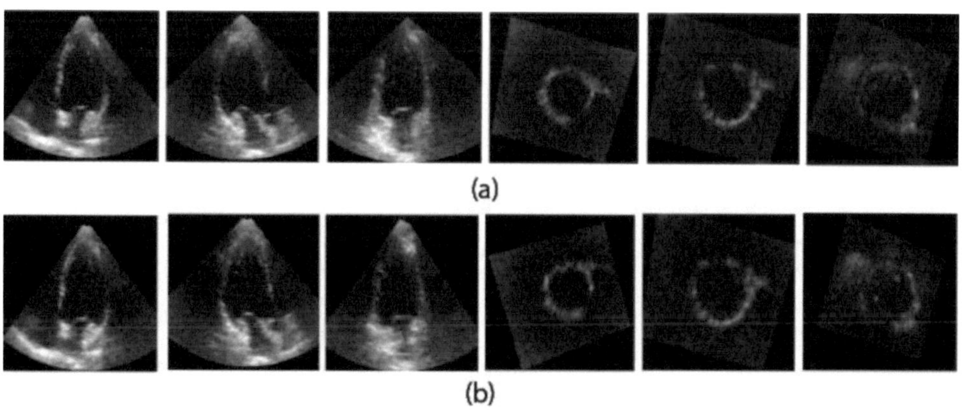

Figure 5. Examples of standard plane extraction, from left to right: A4C, A3C, A2C, PSX AP, PSX PM, and PSX MV: (a) plane extraction results and (b) ground-truth.

normal vector of the ground-truth plane and that of the extracted plane. The distance error is defined as the distance of an anchor on one plane to the other plane, where the anchor is the LV centre. Evaluation results of the proposed method and the previous works by Lu et al. and Chykeyuk et al. [5, 7] are listed in **Table 1**. Average angle errors and distance errors of plane extraction were measured. Run time was measured as the total computational time of the six-plane extraction. The experiments were performed on an Intel® Core™ i7 3.6 GHz computer with 16 GB of RAM. Examples of standard plane extraction are shown in **Figure 5**. As shown in **Table 1**, plane extraction accuracy was improved by about 30%, while computational time was significantly reduced.

3. Automatic foetal weight measurement

3.1. Overview

Generally, growth diagnosis of foetus is used by length of foetal head, abdomen and femur in ultrasound image. Nowadays, it is measured by doctor or clinical examiner, and the measurement process is very complex and needs a long time. In this chapter, a fully automated method for estimated foetal weight (EFW) measurement is proposed. In **Figure 6**, measurement plane images and measurement positions in common ultrasound scanning are shown [12]. Biparietal diameter (BPD) for foetal head, abdominal circumference (AC) for foetal abdomen and femur length (FL) for foetal femur are measured. Using the above three measurement results, foetal weight can be estimated by common formulas such as.

$$\mathrm{EFW} = 1.07 \times \mathrm{BPD}^3 + 0.30 \times \mathrm{AC}^2 \times \mathrm{FL} \tag{4}$$

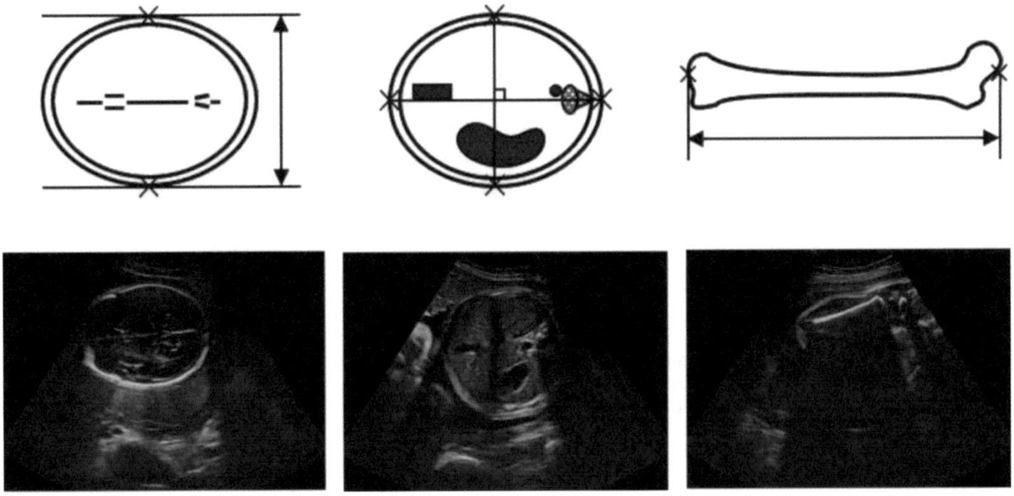

Figure 6. Measurement of foetus (Left: BPD, Mid: AC, Right: FL) [12].

http://dx.doi.org/10.5772/intechopen.76284

3.2. Automatic BPD measurement

In **Figure 7**, the procedures of BPD measurement are shown. At first, the input ultrasound image of the foetal head is transformed to that of polar coordinates, as shown in **Figure 8**. Second, line-route searching on pixels with high intensity in the polar transformed image is performed by using dynamic programming (DP). Third, the detected line route is transformed back to the original image coordinates. Then, ellipse fitting is performed on pixels with high intensity. Here, direct least squares fitting (DLSF) [13] is applied. According to the shape of foetal head, only the ellipses with aspect rates of higher than 0.65 are adopted as candidate results. Next, mid-line of foetal head is masked out, and outer-inner processing is performed to obtain the final BPD measurement result. **Figure 9** shows example results of ellipse fitting and BPD measurement.

3.3. Automatic FL measurement

In **Figure 10**, the procedures of FL measurement are shown. First, as image preprocessing, intensity normalization and weighting is performed to prevent misdetection of tissues of placenta or uterine wall. Second, candidate areas of foetal femur are detected by using entropy binarization [14]. **Figure 11(a)** and **(b)** shows example results of such detected areas. Third, area integration process is performed to extract appropriate range of femur area by using second moment of the candidate area. **Figure 11(c)** shows the integration result of the candidate detected areas in **Figure 11(b)**. Finally, measurement points are detected by intersection points between searching line along the second moment angle and the femur area. **Figure 12** shows the detection result of measurement.

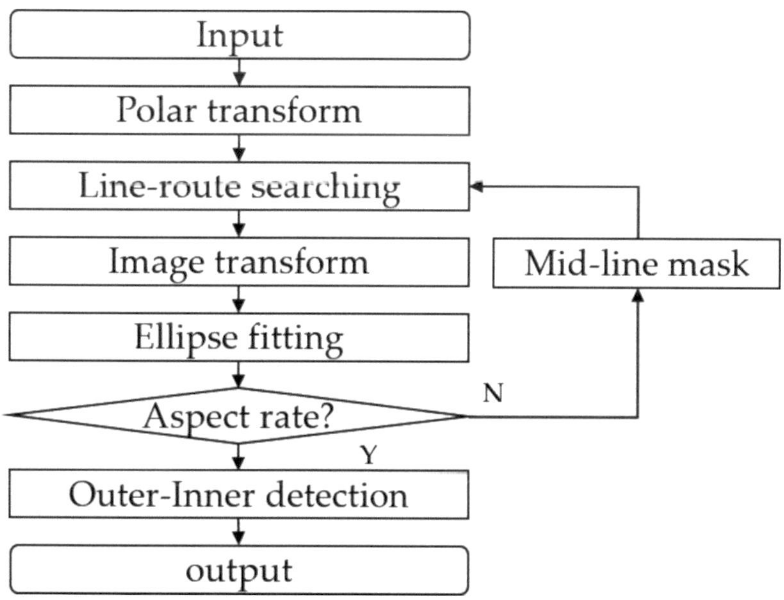

Figure 7. Procedures of BPD measurement.

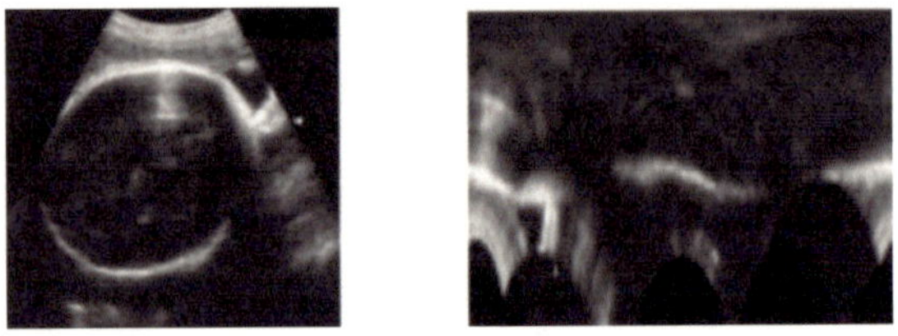

Figure 8. Input image and polar transformed image.

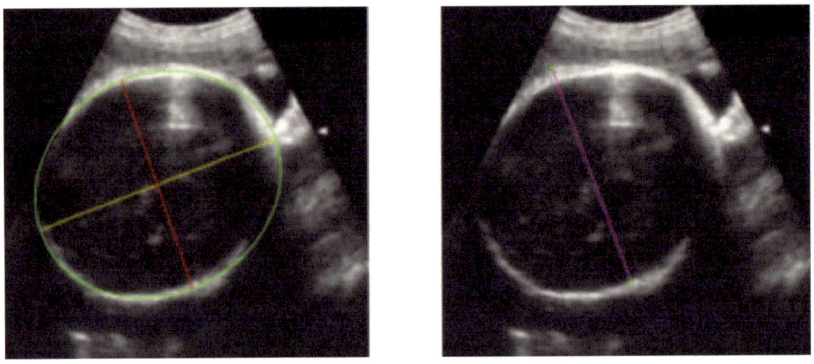

Figure 9. Example results of ellipse fitting (left) and BPD measurement (right).

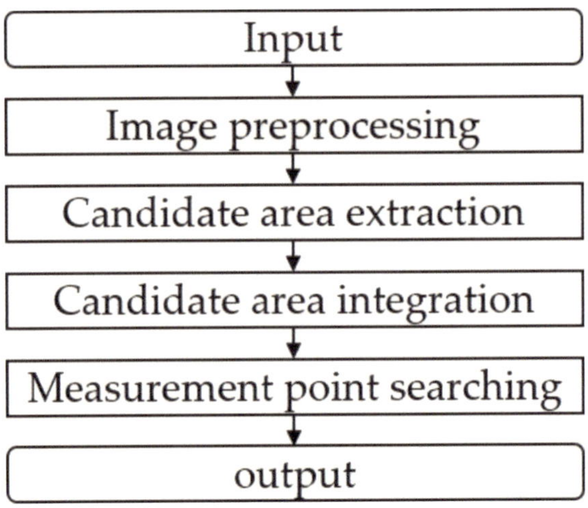

Figure 10. Procedures of FL measurement.

3.4. Automatic AC measurement

In **Figure 13**, the procedures of AC measurement are shown. First, foetal abdomen area is detected by using an AdaBoost classifier. Detection scale is set as 150-500 pixels. Second, feature points representing abdomen contour are extracted by using Laplacian of Gaussian (LoG) filter. Third, ellipse fitting on the abdomen contour candidates is performed. Next, outliers are

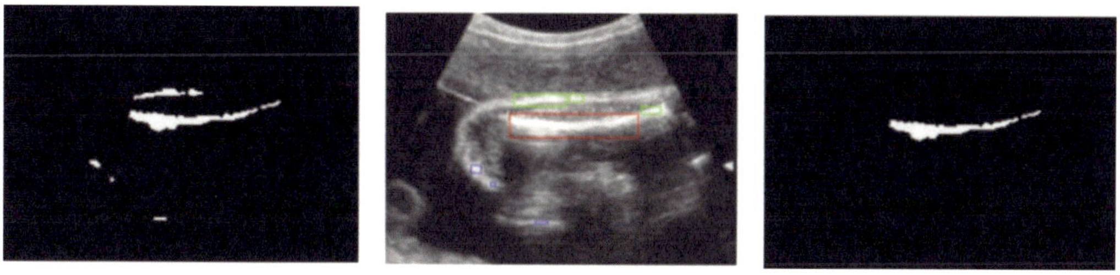

Figure 11. Results of detection: (a) binary image; (b) candidate area; (c) integration result.

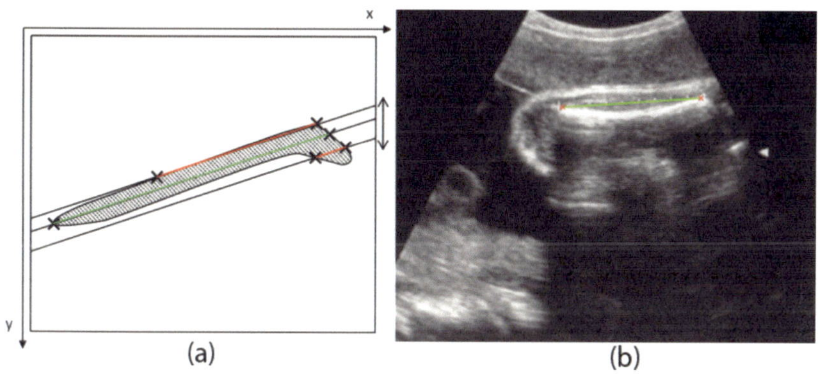

Figure 12. Retection result of FL measurement. (a) Measurement points detection of FL and (b) FL measurement result.

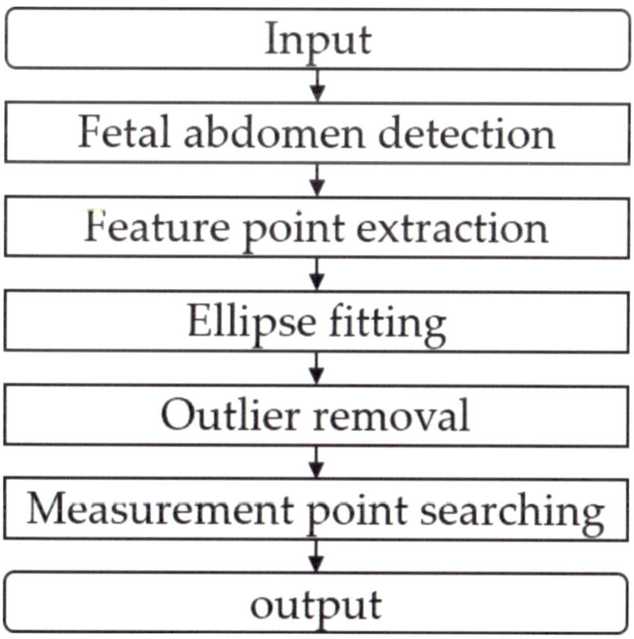

Figure 13. Procedures of AC measurement.

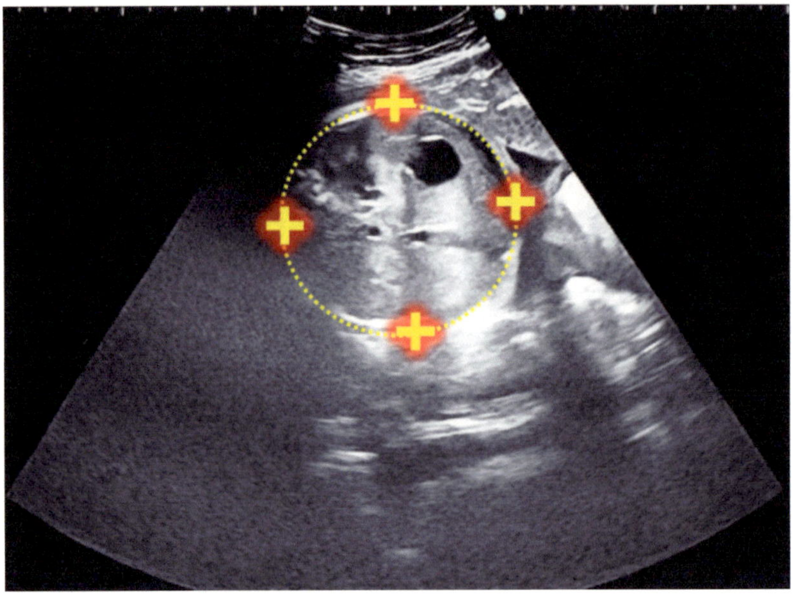

Figure 14. Example of AC measurement points.

	BPD	FL	AC
Success rate (%)	90.6	90.9	93
Run time (ms)	34	5	79

Table 2. Comparison of point detection between Hough forest and proposed method.

removed by using a [15] RANdom Sample Consensus (RANSAC-)based method. Finally, measurement points are detected. **Figure 14** shows an example of obtained measurement points.

3.5. Experiments and discussion

In evaluation experiments, 32 foetal head images, 44 foetal femur images and 105 foetal abdomen images are collected. Measurement points for BPD, FL and AC are automatically detected by using the proposed method. Such results are compared with those of manual measurement. Success rate of measurement and running time (estimate running time in C++) are shown in **Table 2**. We can see that measurement points for foetal weight estimation can be automatically and accurately detected with the proposed method.

4. Ultrasound-CT liver image registration

4.1. Overview

The registration of intraoperative ultrasound image to preoperative planning data is an important issue in the area of surgery navigation. In this chapter, a fully automatic method for anatomical landmark localization, portal vein region classification and intraoperative-preoperative image registration is proposed. The registration framework is shown in **Figure 15**, and the system configuration is shown in **Figure 16**. Before registration, a 3D freehand ultrasound image is acquired with an ultrasound probe which can be tracked by a position sensor. In order to find an appropriate initialization to guide the registration, a specified vessel branch (here, the right and left portal vein branch, PB, is used) is recognized and localized from the ultrasound image and CT image, respectively. The branch localization is based on a Hough forest detector. Then, local 3D images around the detected branches are then extracted from the ultrasound image and CT image, respectively. These two local images are used for the following registration. As a result, a reliable initialization (translation) of the registration is achieved. Next, vessel candidate regions are extracted from both local images. According to the opinions of surgeons, portal vein regions should be used for ultrasound-CT liver image registration. Here, an AdaBoost-based method was proposed for recognizing the portal vein region. Since the coordinates of the extracted portal vein regions can be represented as point sets in 3D space, the vessel point sets of the ultrasound-CT local images are then registered by using iterative closest point (ICP) [16].

4.2. Portal vein branch localization

Hough forest detector mentioned in Section 2.2.1 is modified and applied for the portal vein branch localization. Hough forest provides a way to map from local image patches to anatomical locations. It is a combination of random forest and Hough transform. Hough forests are sets of decision trees learnt from the training data. Each tree in the Hough forest maps local appearance and anatomical locations of image patches to its leaves and each leaf provides a probabilistic vote in the Hough space.

4.3. Vessel candidate region extraction

When the vessel branch is detected, a local 3D image around the branch is cropped from the ultrasound image, and the voxel spacing is resized to $1.0 \times 1.0 \times 1.0$ mm^3. Vessel regions are then extracted from these local images. For the purpose of reducing computational time, a 2D image filtering and thresholding approach is applied. First, 2D image slices are extracted from the ultrasound volume. Then denoise processing by using median filter is executed.

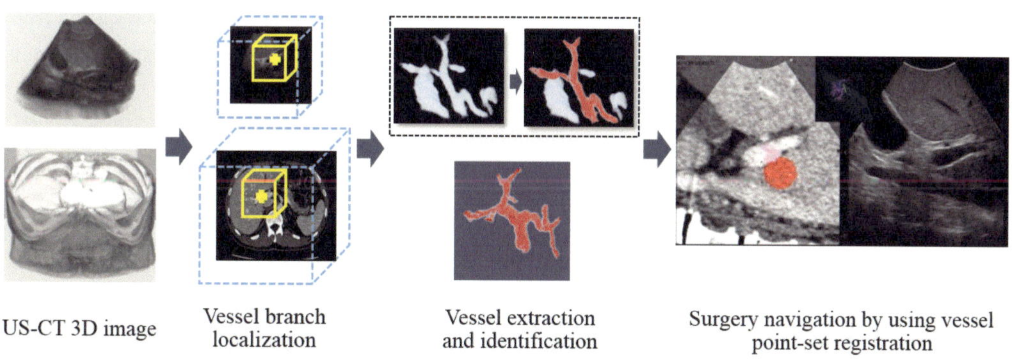

Figure 15. Registration framework.

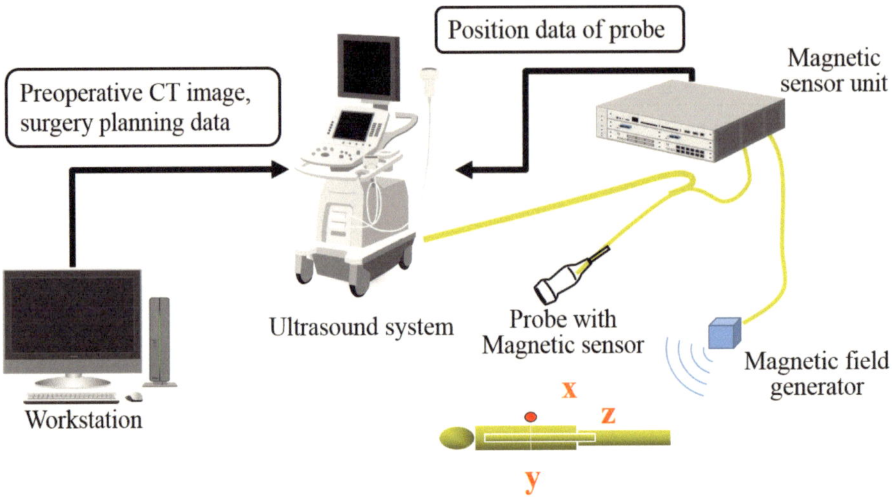

Figure 16. System configuration.

Next, image contrast enhancement is performed, and vessel candidate regions are segmented and binarized on each slice by using an adaptive mean filter. After that, the resulting binary images are constructed to a 3D binary volume. Finally, connected components which include the location of the detected bifurcation are extracted as vessel regions. Brief explanations of the image filtering and thresholding will be given as follows.

Contrast-enhanced filtering: A contrast-enhanced filter is applied to the 2D ultrasound slices as a preprocessing step of the vessel extraction. The filter is defined as:

$$I_{\mathrm{E}} = (I_{\mathrm{M}} - I_{\mathrm{W}}) * k + I_{\mathrm{M}}, \tag{5}$$

where I_{E} is the contrast-enhanced image, I_{M} is a mean-filtered image, I_{W} is a weighted mean-filtered image and k is a coefficient that represents the degree of image contrast enhancement. Here, a 3×3 mean filter and a 3×3 Gaussian filter are used for the mean filtering and the weighted-mean filtering. Coefficient k is set as 2.0 experimentally.

Adaptive mean thresholding: After the contrast-enhanced filtering, image thresholding is applied to the 2D ultrasound images. If the intensity of an interesting pixel is smaller than the threshold value, the pixel is considered as a part of the vessel. Such a threshold value is determined by mean filtering on the local surrounding region of the pixel:

$$v_{\mathrm{th}} = \mu_N - c. \tag{6}$$

Here, μ_N is the output value of an $N \times N$ mean filtering and c is a coefficient that represents the standard deviation of the filtered region. In this work, $N = 5$ and $c = 7$ are determined empirically. The resulting binary images are then reconstructed to a 3D binary image. Since the portal vein volumes are considered to have relative large capacities in liver vessels, only eight of largest labelled volumes are extracted as candidate regions for the next procedure.

4.4. Portal vein region classification

As mentioned earlier, it is necessary to classify and extract portal vein regions from the above vessel candidate regions. In this chapter, a machine learning-based method is proposed for the portal vein region extraction, as shown in **Figure 17**. It is based on an object detector by using AdaBoost classifier [17]. **Figure 18** shows procedures of the proposed method. First, input vessel candidate regions. Second, randomly sample a number of image patches from the input candidate regions. Next, input the image patches to the AdaBoost classifier and perform detection of portal vein objects. Finally, according to the votes of detected portal vein objects, determine whether the vessel candidate regions belong to portal vein.

The AdaBoost classifier is composed of a set of weak learners with associated weights. Each weak learner uses a single image feature to produce a hypothesis. In training process, AdaBoost is used to find the best weak learners and the corresponding weights for these classifiers. In this chapter, portal vein objects are detected from image patches which are randomly sampled from the extracted vessel candidate regions. **Figure 19(a)** shows how the image patches are sampled for training data generation, and **Figure 19(b)** shows some examples of positive and negative image patches. Positive examples are sampled from the extracted regions which belong to portal vein, and negative examples are sampled from other extracted regions which do not belong to portal vein.

In the stage of portal vein region identification, image patches are randomly sampled from five of the largest vessel candidate volumes. The number of image patches sampled from each vessel candidate volume is the same. Next, such image samples are inputs to the trained AdaBoost-based portal vein object detector. Once more than one object of portal vein regions is detected, the image patch is identified as a portal vein sub-region. The number of detected sub-regions is measured on each vessel candidate volume. If this number exceeds a threshold value, the corresponding candidate volume is classified as a portal vein object. The resulted regions are used for ultrasound-CT point-set registration.

4.5. ICP registration of vessel point sets

Since image quality and characteristics of the ultrasound volumes differ greatly from those of preoperative modalities, intensity-based approaches are difficult to obtain a reliable registration

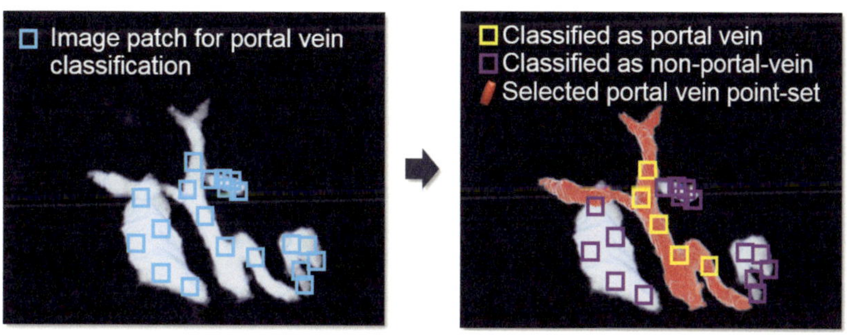

Figure 17. Overview of portal vein region classification.

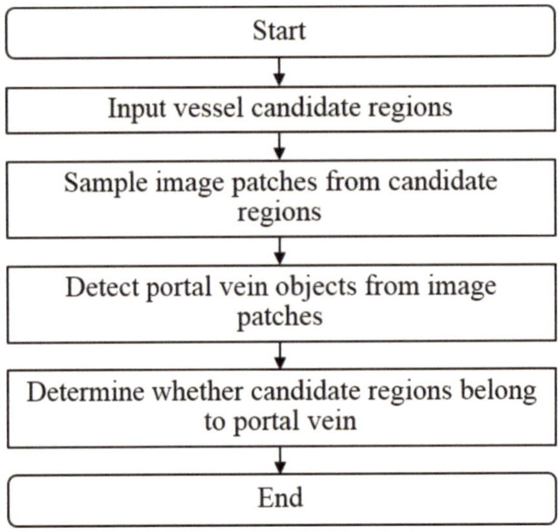

Figure 18. Procedures of portal vein classification.

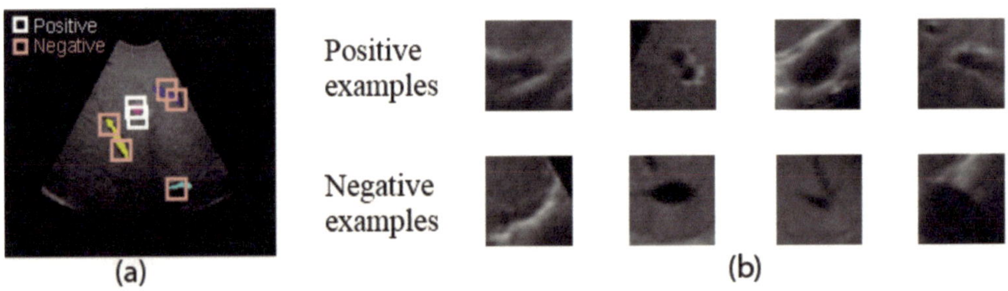

Figure 19. Examples of image patches for training. (a) Image patch sampling and (b) examples of image patches.

result. On the other hand, coordinates of the segmented vessel regions can be considered as point sets in 3D space. Such point sets without intensity information are able to be utilized to a registration. Here, ICP method for point set registration is applied. **Figure 20** illustrates an example of ultrasound-CT vessel point-set registration; the first row shows the point sets and the second row shows the corresponding cross-sections of CT and ultrasound images. For initial registration, a large scale of transformation is needed to be estimated. Fortunately, only rotation should be updated since vessel branch detection already provides rough translation. For the fine registration, a robust method of wrong-pair rejection is applied for removing vessel points outside the field of view (FOV) of an ultrasound image.

4.6. Experiments and discussion

Ultrasound-CT image registration accuracy was evaluated by using clinical data acquired in liver resection surgery. Ultrasound-CT images from 44 patients were used in the experiment.

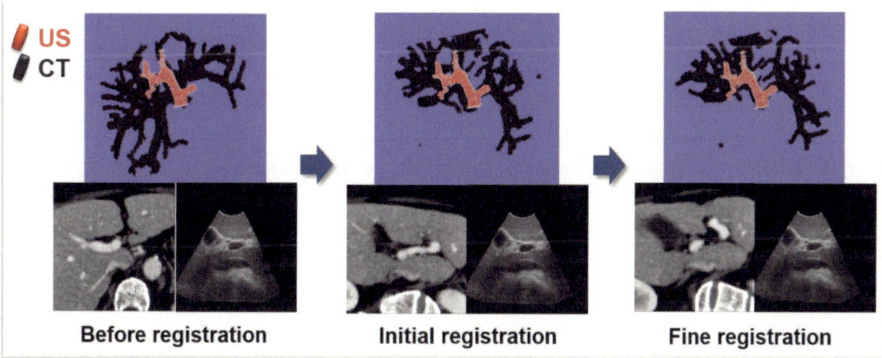

Figure 20. An example of US-CT point-set registration.

Since more than 1 ultrasound volume is acquired from each patient, 30 CT images and 114 ultrasound images of 30 patients were for training, and 14 CT images and 36 ultrasound images of 14 patients were for testing. Dimension sizes of the CT and ultrasound images are $512 \times 512 \times (134\text{~}231)$ and $448 \times 448 \times (89\text{~}192)$, respectively. Image resolutions are $0.683 \times 0.683 \times (1\text{~}1.5)$ mm^3 and $(0.328\text{~}0.46987) \times (0.328\text{~}0.46987) \times (0.719\text{~}1.226)$ mm^3, respectively. All the experiments were performed on a system with Intel® Core™ i7 CPU 3.70-GHz and 12-GB memory. Evaluation results are shown in **Table 3**. The proposed method was compared with our previous work [2]. In [2], we set a searching area around the branch, set sample points inside the area and estimate and threshold the vesselness by using Hessian-based filtering. The connected region with the largest number of vessel points is considered as portal vein region. Registration that has an error less than 30 mm is considered as a succeeded one. Distance between the measurement points before registration was 137.6 ± 18.1 mm. After registration, errors of the proposed method and our previous work were 8.7 ± 4.4 and 10.2 ± 8.7 mm, respectively. Success rates were 94.4 and 77.8%, respectively. Running time of the proposed method was 9.3 s and that of the previous work was 8.1 s. It can be seen that the proposed method outperforms the previous work by improving both the registration accuracy and robustness. The running time is slightly longer than that of the previous work because AdaBoost-based classification is performed to select portal vein regions. The objectives of registration error, success rate and running time were achieved. The study was approved by the ethics committee of Hitachi group headquarters.

	Distance before registration (mm)	Registration error (mm)	Success rate (error < 30 mm)	Running time (s)
Proposed method	137.6 ± 18.1	8.7 ± 4.4	34/36 = 94.4%	9.3
Previous work [2]		10.2 ± 8.7	28/36 = 77.8%	8.1

Table 3. Comparison of point detection between Hough forest and proposed method.

5. Conclusion

Fully automatic techniques for ultrasound imaging applications of cardiac plane extraction, foetal weight measurement and ultrasound-CT image registration for liver surgery navigation are introduced. With such techniques, automatic ultrasound examination and navigation can be achieved accurately and efficiently. Workflow in diagnosis and treatment by using ultrasound image analysis can be improved.

Author details

Zisheng Li*, Peifei Zhu, Takashi Toyomura and Yoshimi Noguchi

*Address all correspondence to: zisheng.li.fj@hitachi.com

Hitachi, Ltd., Tokyo, Japan

References

[1] Zhu P, Li Z. Guideline-based machine learning for standard plane extraction in 3D cardiac ultrasound. In: Proceedings of Medical Computer Vision and Bayesian and Graphical Models for Biomedical Imaging (MCV '16), 17-21 October. Athens, Greece: Springer; 2016. pp. 137-147

[2] Li Z, Zhu P. Liver ultrasound portal vein classification for navigation of liver-tumor resection surgery. In: Proceedings of the 31st International Congress and Exhibition (CARS '17), 20-24 June 2017. Barcelona, Spain: Springer; 2017. pp. S101-S102

[3] Li Z, Zhu P, Suzuki M. Anatomical landmark localization and ultrasound-CT image registration applied to surgery navigation of hepatectomy. In: Proceedings of the 30th International Congress and Exhibition (CARS '16), 21-25 June 2016. Heidelberg, Germany: Springer; 2016

[4] Lang RM, Badano LP, et al. Recommendations for cardiac chamber quantification by echocardiography in adults: An update from the American Society of Echocardiography and the European Association of Cardiovascular Imaging. Journal of the American Society of Echocardiography. 2015;**28**(1):1-39. DOI: 10.1016/j.echo.2014.10.003

[5] Lu X, Georgescu B, et al. Automated detection of planes from three-dimensional echocardiographic data. U.S. Patent. No. 8,073,215.6; 2011

[6] Zheng Y, Barbu A, et al. Fast automatic heart chamber segmentation from 3D CT data using marginal space learning and steerable features. In: Proceedings International Conference on Computer Vision (ICCV '07), 14-21 October 2007. Rio de Janeiro Brazil: IEEE; 2007. pp. 1-8

[7] Chykeyuk K, Yaqub M, Noble JA. Class-specific regression random forest for accurate extraction of standard planes from 3d echocardiography. In: Proceedings of International MICCAI Workshop on Medical Computer Vision (MCV '13), 2013. Nogoya, Japan: Springer; 2013. pp. 53-62

[8] Criminisi A, Shotton J, et al. Regression forests for efficient anatomy detection and localization in CT studies. In: Proceedings of International MICCAI Workshop on Medical Computer Vision (MCV '10), 2010. Beijing, China: Springer; 2010. pp. 106-117

[9] Gall J, Lempitsky V. Class-specific Hough forests for object detection. In: Criminisi A, Shotton J, editors. Decision Forests for Computer Vision and Medical Image Analysis. London: Springer; 2013. pp. 143-157. DOI: 10.1007/978-1-4471-4929-3_11

[10] Gall J, Yao A, Razavi N, et al. Hough forests for object detection, tracking, and action recognition. IEEE Transactions on Pattern Analysis and Machine Intelligence. 2011;**33**(11): 2188-2202. DOI: 10.1109/TPAMI.2011.70

[11] Tobon-Gomez C, De Craene M, et al. Benchmarking framework for myocardial tracking and deformation algorithms: An open access database. Journal of Medical Image Analysis. 2013;**17**(6):632-648. DOI: 10.1016/j.media.2013.03.008

[12] Tsustsumi S. Obstetrical ultrasound examination. Journal of Japan Society of Obstetrics and Gynecology. 2010;**62**(7):90-97

[13] Fitzgibbon A, Maurizio P, Robert BF. Direct least square fitting of ellipses. IEEE Transactions on Pattern Analysis and Machine Intelligence. 1999;**21**(5):476-480. DOI: 10.1109/34.765658

[14] Wang C. Automatic entropy-based femur segmentation and fast length measurement for fetal ultrasound images. In: Proceedings of Advanced Robotics and Intelligent Systems (ARIS '14), 6-8 June 2014. Taiwan: IEEE; 2014. pp. 1-5

[15] Fischler MA, Bolles RC. Random sample consensus: A paradigm for model fitting with applications to image analysis and automated cartography. Journal of Communications of the ACM. 1981;**24**(6):381-395. DOI: 10.1145/358669.358692

[16] Besl PJ, McKay ND. A method for registration of 3-D shapes. IEEE Transactions on Pattern Analysis and Machine Intelligence. 1992;**14**(2):239-256. DOI: 10.1109/34.121791

[17] Ojala T et al. Multiresolution gray-scale and rotation invariant texture classification with local binary patterns. IEEE Transactions on Pattern Analysis and Machine Intelligence. 2002;**24**:971-987. DOI: 10.1109/TPAMI.2002.1017623